EAT
FAT

Also by RICHARD KLEIN

Cigarettes Are Sublime

RICHARD KLEIN

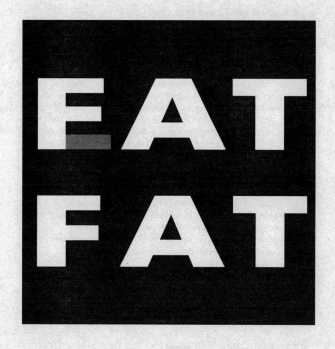

EAT
FAT

PICADOR

First published 1996 by Pantheon, a division of Random House, USA

First published in Great Britain 1997 by Picador

This edition published 1997 by Picador
an imprint of Macmillan Publishers Ltd
25 Eccleston Place London SW1W 9NF
and Basingstoke

Associated companies throughout the world

ISBN 0 330 34294 0

· *Grateful acknowledgement is made to the following for permission to reprint previously
published material*: *C. M. Donald*: Excerpt from *The Fat Woman Measures Up* by C. M. Donald
(Ragweed Press, Charlottetown, Prince Edward Island, C1A 7N7 Canada). Copyright © 1986
by C. M. Donald. Reprinted by permission of C. M. Donald – *Duke University Press*: Excerpt
from *Fat Art, Thin Art* by Eve Kosovsky Sedgwick. Copyright © 1994 by Duke University Press.
Reprinted by permission of Duke University Press, Durham, NC.

Book Design by M. Kristen Bearse

9 8 7 6 5 4 3 2 1

A CIP catalogue record for this book is available
from the British Library.

Printed and bound in Great Britain
Mackays of Chatham plc, Chatham, Kent

A TAMARA

CONTENTS

ACKNOWLEDGMENTS

I feel so strongly that this book is a collaborative effort that I don't
have the right merely to acknowledge those whose work this truly
is. I have mostly been a scribe, collecting and collating ideas and
dreams about fat that have been fed to me by a lot of people living
and dead. It is the living I want to acknowledge first. Their inter-
ventions and contributions came at such decisive and opportune
moments that I began to feel even more strongly the power of a collective idea shaping itself in my mind, under my hands.

David Shipley at the *New Republic* first evoked the idea of
turning my attention to fat, and he collaborated generously in writing the earliest sketch. To have had the privilege of his editorial
attention transformed my own relationship to writing.

Kim Witherspoon, my agent, is a great and heroic reader,
whose powerful enthusiasms lent me confidence to write this

ACKNOWLEDGMENTS

book. Her laser realism spared me many pitfalls. Maria Massie, her associate, shares the credit. So, in England, does Abner Stein.

My editor, Erroll McDonald, a wise and thoughtful man, has a miraculous capacity to put himself inside your head and think your thoughts better than you can, in view of a book. His conceptions and his understanding are reflected everywhere in these pages.

Nara Nahm, at Pantheon, did the heavy lifting with me, with infallible intelligence, perfect taste, and a rugged work ethic. My wonderful daughter-in-law, Debra Helfand, also at Random House, corrected my prose and organized my thoughts.

My English publisher, Jonathan Riley, lavishly gave me the benefit of his perfect literary judgment and his uncanny appreciation of prose. Alyson Menzies, at Picador, spent days teaching me about making books and eating fat.

At Cornell, my colleague Professor David Levitsky, working together with Terri Garrison, inspired my earliest thinking with the force of their extraordinary work on behalf of fat acceptance. They are testimony to the ways that seriously meditating on fat enriches one's moral life and stirs political passion to action. In addition, I owe much to my colleagues and students at Cornell for their encouragement and suggestions.

Judy Bronstein, in Sarasota, by her active, personal interest in this work, contributed to many of its ideas and formulations; she brought to it an engaged feminine perspective, which powerfully influenced the whole tone and stance of the book. Jan Holmes and Dwight Hoover lent me the advantage of their political intelligence, their wit, and their incomparable loyalty.

I beg forgiveness from my sister, from my mother, for the use I make of them in these pages, and thank my father for his patience and his martinis. I'm most of all grateful for Jonah, my main man.

Finally, this book reflects the taste and embodies the work of Tamara Parker, as much as it does mine. She has been present at every stage of its elaboration, and has written or rewritten, or corrected or approved every sentence here. She has been its *sine qua non*, she without whose encyclopedic brilliance and critical taste this book,

       EAT

       FAT, would not be.

She, in turn, would have asked me to say that she owes much to Telumé.

A PREFACE IN CONCLUSION

SKIP THIS PREFACE!

This preface is written for people who want to know what they're getting into. I have a lot of sympathy for people like that, who want to be sure in advance that what they're about to do is worth the risk or trouble, or the expense. But I also pity those who won't take the trouble to take the risk of entering on a path whose detours and circling back, whose pleasures and dangers, are entirely unpredictable and slightly alarming. But it's necessary, if this book is to work, that you suspend your need to know in advance where you're going. Reading this preface will probably tell you more than you need to know. As a result, the effect of this book will be lessened and its impact softened. What's in this book should produce its effect more or less unconsciously. It will likely be filtered out and censored by what you learn in advance in this preface.

So don't read this preface, if you want this book to work. Consider it a conclusion, and come back to it.

This book aspires to be something like a mandala, like one of those beautiful geometrical mazes before which Buddhists sit and meditate. In its forms and pathways lie places where the mind returns to think about its own incessant movement. A mandala is the symbol of a lifelong struggle of the self with the self to overcome its compulsions, repetitions, and blocks. Carl Jung, the celebrated analyst, spent his adult life building his own house like a mandala, constantly adding to it and changing its walls in an ongoing process of constructing around himself, while inhabiting, his most primitive dreams and elemental desires.

The medium of this mandala is fat. For me, as it has been for my mother and my sister, fat has been the focus of a constant, daily preoccupation. In front of any mirror or in the mind's eye. Every day of our lives, it has been the object of a little mantra in which we recite the story of who we think we are, how we feel about ourselves, what we want for our lives in the future.

This book aims to be a sort of meditation object over which one reflects with the view of effecting a change. Its aim is to focus intensely on fat in order to quiet the mind of fat obsession, and to liberate the self from its compulsions, with consequences that are hard to predict.

You will note a certain repetitive intonation in the style of this book. It is intentionally intended to serve the same subterranean effect as prayer, which achieves its liberations through repetition. If it succeeds, it works like prayer to engender a repeating rhythm that frees the mind from its infinite distractions and allows other thoughts to form.

Without being maniacal, I've tried to write this book using the shortest words I could, as if every word in this book was trying to be the one word, the same word, fat. It is as if you could stop obsessing about fat if you could simply be repeating over and over again at every moment, like a little tune beneath your consciousness, that single word: FAT.

My mother, my sister, and I have been preoccupied with fat most of our lives, most of our adult lives. So has my father, who is very thin; he's had to deal with our dealing with fat. For us, it has been a perpetual source of preoccupation and self-regard, the origin of some of our most negative feelings about ourselves and despair about our chances. There have been times when I have thought that our family obsession was a great loss, of time and energy and focus. But as I've been thinking and writing about fat for several years, I've grown to appreciate the intellectual and personal value that this family reflection on fat has acquired. The fat we ponder serves to embody our hungers, visibly manifests the power of our cravings, the drive for satisfaction and the urge to pleasure, as well as much that is self-destructive, self-demeaning in our lives. Our characters have been shaped by our fat and by our attitude toward it. In America, at the end of the twentieth century, it has been for us, as for many others, the most sustained focus of our concerned attention, the single most important material object of meditation in our lives.

Even more serious, of course, are those for whom fat has become a matter of life and death. Either because they have too much or too little of it. There is unmistakable evidence of the implication of fat in increasing risk of heart disease and diabetes. For many, victims of heart attacks, the low-fat diets of doctors like Dean Ornish have saved their lives. Reducing the amount of fat in your diet down to 10 percent or less, as is recommended for many heart patients, can have dramatic benefits for improving or stabilizing one's condition. This book does not pretend otherwise. But for the vast majority of people the risks of what is called obesity have to be measured against the risks entailed in combating it. Diets can kill, and yo-yo dieting has specific and long-term health implications that need to be weighed against the risks of being "overweight."

The medical risk of obesity, this book aims to suggest, has been severely overstated. For reasons that are often misguided or venal, doctors and nutritionists skew their studies to reflect their biases or wishes. A recent study by one of the most severe anti-fat nutritionists will allow us to see how relatively small are the risks for most people, how they compare with the risks of dieting, and how easily the risk can be manipulated by scientists and nutritionists, by health and fitness experts to prove what it is in their interest to prove. The diet industry alone, with its products and services, generates over 30 billion dollars a year of the American economy. Imminent future developments in pharmaceuticals, in new diet drugs, could raise even that figure substantially. As we will see, the stakes are enormous in persuading people that even small amounts of fat increase their risk of early death. Particularly now, at a moment when it has become clear that diets don't work, new drugs are being introduced whose dangers to public health are minimized by persuading people of their risk at being even slightly overweight. For if the public and the FDA can be persuaded that even a little fat is dangerous, and that diets don't work, then the only solution to this dilemma is drugs. They are the American solution for everything.

Baba Ram Dass, once known as Richard Alpert, was one of the early experimentors with LSD. He and Timothy Leary did the first clinical trials in the psychology department at Harvard, until Harvard threw them out, worried about the scientific character of the marathon trips they were sponsoring, using large and larger doses of the purest possible acid. Alpert, his mind blown or elevated, went to India to seek his guru. After traveling around the subcontinent with a holy man from Malibu, he found his very guru. He was a little old man, wrapped in a blanket, on the top of a mountain, surrounded by a few devotees in attendance. Alpert knew this was his guru, because the man could read his mind. He looked at Alpert and uttered the word "Mother." Alpert's mother had just died of stomach cancer. Then, with no words having been exchanged, the guru added, "Large in the stomach."

After a while, Alpert gave his guru an enormous dose of the very pure Harvard acid he was carrying. He wanted to observe the effect it would have on this already very high, very spiritual man. He also hoped that the guru would enlighten him about the nature and value of the states induced by the drug. He also thought it would help him understand the guru's drug-free elevation. The guru took the dose and sat impassively, wrapped in his blanket, seemingly oblivious to its effects, except for his prolonged silence. The effects of LSD increase as one ages, and the guru's first dose was massive. After eight hours, having come down, he turned to Alpert and said, "This is the avatar of the Americans." Alpert, or Baba Ram Dass, understood this to mean that for God to appear to

Americans, He had to assume the form of a drug. Ours is such a materialist culture that divinity can manifest itself to us only in the form of a pharmaceutical substance. By the same logic, any antidote we find to counteract the power of evil in us must assume the form of a pill. Anorexants, anti-fat drugs, are like a chemical exorcism, the silver bullet that will kill the vampire of our fat.

Behind the hideous mask of demon fat is a beauty that this book aims to recall. Beautiful fat bodies are on display here; their charms and seduction, as they are represented in art or in pornography are attentively explored. For most of the history of art, artists have loved fat bodies; in the history of cooking, fat has had a starring role. The only recipes in this book are those for the most fattening dishes imaginable, at least to me, who loves to imagine them.

Fat is beautiful, sexy, and strong. Politicians cultivate it, singers require it, gourmets appreciate it, and lovers play with it. *Fat* is a fabulous three-letter word.

LIST OF ILLUSTRATIONS

EAT
FAT

INTRO-DUCTION

You have a choice of titles for this book. You could call it *Fat Fat*. One reason for that title arises from the fact that there is something about the word itself, in its long history, that has always made people want to say it twice. It's been true at least since Shakespeare. "Wits they have; gross, gross; fat, fat," says Rosaline in *Love's Labour's Lost* (V, ii, 267). Sometimes the desire to repeat the word emerges in the frequent use of F-words to accompany fat: as in fat fellow, fat fool, fat friend, fat friar, feed fat, fat with feasting, fat and fulsome, fat Falstaff, to cite only some Shakespearean examples. It's as if the word itself is always wanting to double itself, or f-f-f-f-at, to stutter in order to expand itself, to grow itself fatter as a word, already a little tub. That's also why Olestra, a new synthetic oil that can be used in cooking, quickly gets called fake fat, or fat-free fat.

3

But the title is also a way of pointing up the importance this book attaches to the difference between fat and fat—between the adjective and the noun. If the noun, the substantive fat, on your hips or on your lips, is generally viewed negatively these days, the adjective can still be used with its older connotations, when it attributed positive value to things. After all, something that has the virtue of being fat can still, for example, be rich and fertile, like fat soil or a fat check. It can even be cute and cuddly, like a fat baby or a fat chick. This is a book about fat fat.

But you've noticed by the way the title is printed on the jacket cover that you can also read it EAT

FAT.

You can see how easily EAT turns into FAT just by making something vanish (like food or a line). The point is: this is a postmodern diet book. Postmodern, in my personal dictionary, refers to the contemporary experience of immaterial realities. That is why, in the first place, this book is designed to be thrown away. Once you have consumed it, the text should vanish, and remain only a delicious memory, like the faint recurrence of the feeling of well-being that accompanies the disappearance into your mouth of a golden chocolate truffle. But save the jacket. Cut it out and paste it on your fridge if you want this book to go on working. Once you've read it, all you really need for the book to work again is to remember the sign for it, *Fat Fat*, or see its title, EAT

FAT.

I'll explain. Most of the signs you see on refrigerator doors try to coax, scold, or tease you into eating thin—into "watching" what you eat. You can judge their success by consulting your personal experience or the latest statistical evidence. According to the most recent measurements, Americans as a whole are about 10 percent fatter than they were twelve years ago. That's true for men and women, children and adults, the elderly and teenagers. Anecdotal as well as demographic evidence confirms the fact: currently, we are getting fatter faster. The same is true in Britain and Spain, Japan and France, but especially here in America, already perhaps the fattest nation in a world itself growing increasingly fat. (Despite some famines.)

Why this should be so at this moment in history is a mystery. A mystery of history. We ought to be growing in the opposite direction—growing thin. For more than forty years—more intensely in the last twenty—the health-beauty-fitness industry has mobilized immense resources of wealth and creativity to persuade us of the virtues of skinny. Last year alone consumers spent $33 billion on weight loss, with largely negative results. Morbid obesity has skyrocketed in the last seven years (officially, it's morbid when you are 40 pounds over your ideal weight). The latest statistics indicate that the number of overweight children has more than doubled in the last thirty years.[*] In Britain, 50 percent of adults are overweight.[†] As a whole we're getting fatter. Something appears to be very wrong.

But rather than regret this trend, as many with alarm so often do, we ought for a moment to consider that what is actually happening might just have some good reason to happen. Perhaps we

[*] *New York Times,* October 11, 1995.
[†] *The Economist,* September 30, 1995.

are all supposed to be getting fatter, since that's what we're doing anyway, despite all our efforts to the contrary.

This book proceeds on the assumption that what *is* has a very strong claim on being what is supposed to be. It's hard to believe there isn't some necessity, some evolutionary requirement or social logic, that explains what is taking place. Otherwise, why are we so rapidly accomplishing the opposite of what we are trying so urgently to achieve? It is everywhere assumed that, getting fat, we have lost control, and that by exercising more of it, we will become what we should be, instead of what we are mostly fast becoming— fat. It is endlessly repeated: We eat too much and don't exercise enough. It always comes down and gets back to that. All the diet books, all the diagnoses and prescriptions ultimately spring from a single idea, the same principle, endlessly repeated like a mantra: Calories ingested, calories expended. They all conclude with the same advice: eat less, move more. And so people take control; they start to diet and they take up physical exercise, and within three or four years 95 percent of them are even fatter.

But just for a moment assume that it is no accident, that there are unavoidable biological or ecological constraints, resistless forces, sociological or psychological, inexorably requiring, as a matter of fact, that at this moment in history we damn well ought to be getting fatter. Maybe there's some evolutionary necessity secretly at work to make us fat. Maybe fat will decrease our chances of developing some disease in the future or protect us against imminent dangers in the environment—like food scarcity or undiscovered toxins. Perhaps there are general cultural trends that we have only begun to suspect, historical cycles of fat and thin, which correspond to different stages of history or stages, say, in the development of capitalism. It has been proposed that people are fatter in periods of accelerated capital formation, when wealth is being rapidly accumulated. Perhaps it's the spirit of the times, a moment in some long cycle of fat years and lean, linked to moments in the history of human spirituality, when the body is alternately starved or indulged. The asceticism of the Romantic period, which aspired to be otherworldly, made fashionable an ethereal look. It fostered a certain idea of slim beauty, not seen in Europe since the Gothic Middle Ages, that contrasted starkly with both the exuberantly plump ideal of the eighteenth-century aristocracy and the idea of beauty favored at the end of the nineteenth century in Europe and America, which was fat.

Why now? Why more than ever do people have fat on their minds, while adding it to their hips? Perhaps today, moving less and getting fatter are the inevitable consequences of living surrounded by video screens. *Surrounded* may not be the word—invaded, incorporated, absorbed by video screens is what we seem increasingly to be. The virtual lives we lead in front of screens, in cyberspace, are, more than ever, the only lives we get. Is it any wonder, as virtual reality becomes more our only reality, that muscle and bone lose much of their traditional utility and our bodies get generally fatter? Work and play take the physical form of immobile contemplation in front of a screen, with the mind perfectly absorbed, while the body remains still. Remember that Buddha, too, was fat.

People are always blaming fat on television. Other explanations are plausible. Maybe the approach of the end of the millennium arouses simultaneously inordinate anxieties and a spirit of jubilation. New Year's Eve, when you ordinarily celebrate to mask your disquiet, is a time of socially sanctioned transition. We eat too much, drink and make loud noises, to conceal from ourselves the arbitrary limits of time and the finitude of our lives, to which transitions attest. But today, what is about to expire is a millennium, and on the horizon dawns not just another century but a New Order, we hope—and fear. A thousand years, perhaps, of human civilization—starting with us. What better to do than to eat?

In the temporal passing between the end of the old and the start of the new year, between one millennium and another, there is an instant that belongs to neither—a transitory moment out of time that makes it possible to mark the moment of passage from one dated instant to another. The arbitrary and fateful fact of that universally acknowledged moment—that time out of time—reminds us of death, our own. After all, the only date that has more importance for the world than the turn of the millennium, we think, is the date of our own death. It's not too soon to start eating.

In these gay nineties, as the millennium approaches, banqueting will once again begin to flourish and feasting to abound. It's an old story. Two thousand years ago Jesus promised banquets for the new millennium: "And I appoint unto you a kingdom . . . that ye may eat and drink at my table in my kingdom." (Luke 22:29–30) In Burgundy and Flanders a thousand years ago, false prophets, like Eudes and Tanchelm—hallucinating heretics who thought they were the messiah—held splendid ceremonial banquets for their followers, which were supposed to recall the "messianic banquet" that the Gospels foretell.[°]

[°] Norman Cohen, *The Pursuit of the Millennium* (London: Secker and Warburg, 1957), p. 53.

A hundred years ago, in the 1890s, hopes and fears about the transition to a new century gave rise to the so-called Banquet Years, when no one missed an occasion to celebrate, at interminable banquets with vast quantities of eating and drinking and much pouring out of speeches. Americans in those days were enormously fat. Autopsy revealed that Diamond Jim Brady had a stomach four times as big as the average man's, but his gargantuan and quite abnormal capacity for food became a model to which successful men aspired. He was the paragon of his age, when copper kings and robber barons took pride in the vastness of their appetite and saw their affluence reflected in their paunch. Lillian Russell was admired for the immensity of her appetite. President Taft weighed over three hundred pounds at his inauguration. Magazines gave women directions for adding weight, in order to increase the profusion of their décolleté, flesh billowing up and cascading down over and out of dresses designed to be worn with corsets that pinch the waist and balloon breasts. Books were written with titles like *How to Become Plump*, by T. C. Duncan.

Just as it happened a century ago, we too have become fat at century's end. But instead of celebrating and admiring fat, instead of allowing ourselves the immense and maybe necessary pleasures of eating it and accumulating it, we put signs on our refrigerator directing us to eat thin. Mountains of fat are served every day off greasy grills all over America while we exhort ourselves to cut fat. And the more loudly, and insistently, we execrate its poison and loathe its look, the more we pile it on our plate and add it to our hips.

Maybe we are due for a food crisis like the oil crisis in the 1970s. Maybe for a brief time, in six to nine months, food suddenly will become much harder to get or expensive to buy, because of some environmental fact or political upheaval or some conjunction of events. Suddenly, subtly, the value of fat might change, and once again it would begin to be the case, as it has been so many times before in history, that fat looked good. The rich and the glamorous might once more display their fat, advertising its abundance and their success, in the midst of scarcity.

Perhaps there are many overdetermined reasons why we are bound to be getting fatter. But instead of our celebrating what we are in fact becoming, the shrill voice of skinny is heard across the land, magnified by the chorus of doctors, nutritionists, beauticians, and insurers of all kinds who deplore what we already despise.

Many reasons and diverse motives reinforce our desire to be thin; here are three, widely acknowledged and generally understood.

1. Fat is ugly. Our commitment to a certain slim ideal of human beauty is only about a century old, but it has already become second nature. It has come to seem perfectly natural to hate fat. Even the thin among us dream of dropping five or ten pounds. Losing weight, we imagine, will make us more sexy, productive, and rich. But it's not just the commercial interest and social value we derive from our investment in thin, in a world where fat girls struggle and skinny ones model. Above all, it's our stake in an idea of beauty that compels us to want to be thin and to encourage others—for example, our children—as well. In our eyes—in our mind's eye—we love the look of thin. Fat disgusts.

2. Fat is unhealthy. The medical-nutrition-insurance-beauty industry has for some time promoted the notion that fat kills, that the more drastically we limit it, in our food and on our bodies, the more we increase our chances of longevity. Fat poisons.

3. Fat weighs us down, slows us up. Our progressive need for greater energy and a desire to step more lightly upon the earth seem at odds with fat. Many of those who have written about the history of fat in the twentieth century have seen the connection between the dream of thinness and the modern desire for greater agility, flexibility, and speed. Energy is the principal gain, it is supposed, from being thin, some kinetic enhancement that makes us more vital, more excited, more suited in our bodies for the exhilarations inspired by the modern pleasures of machine speed. This conviction persists despite the evidence, irrefutably accumulated in repeated studies, that fat people are sexier: they want more sex more often than thin people.

Researchers at Michael Reese Hospital in Chicago a few years ago came up with the startling finding that fat women are more sexually appetitive than thinner women. Beller, who first reported this fact, adds that the researchers themselves were surprised, since they had assumed that fat women would be more likely to be frigid, given the greater difficulty they were supposed to have finding partners and the rigid psychic armor that growing fat was supposed to construct. She cites other evidence that obese people are more persevering. The fat are harder to get started than the more easily excited thin, but once they get going they are more difficult to stop. More inertia, she suggests.*

Fat is hot and ready, but thin looks fast and sleek. Fat sucks.

* Anne Scott Beller, *Fat and Thin* (New York: Farrar, Straus & Giroux, 1977), pp. 74–76.

All these reasons or motives to be thin have been challenged in recent years by those who have been seized by the contradiction between what we are and increasingly are becoming and what we are encouraged to desire and to love.

But the hardest work is learning to love fat. It isn't easy, because it really can't be learned. If it ever becomes easy, it will be because one day fashion shifts. We will all wake up one day and just happen to sort of realize that we've started loving the way fat looks. At that moment there will be a sudden change in what we know to be beautiful, without knowing how we know it. Such shifts in taste often occur suddenly, abruptly, as when the Beatles grew their hair long in a moment of vast upheaval, a cultural revolution. But sometimes taste shifts slowly, in a process that feels evolutionary. Where fat is concerned, we have gone so long in an all but uninterrupted progression toward thin that a reversal may be shortly upon us. But don't count on it. It's been predicted before. Hillel Schwartz, the great historian of diets, predicted ten years ago that the growing disparity between our thin ideal and our increasing weight made a shift in the paradigm inevitable and likely to be soon. He was wrong then. Times have changed.

As for the question of health, this book takes as an axiomatic premise the position of Dr. David Levitsky, a nutritionist at Cornell University and one of the heroes of fat acceptance, who notes that "it is hard to let go of the idea that it is always unhealthy to be fat, *even among professionals*" (my italics).* He might have meant,

* Terri Nicholetti Garrison, with David Levitsky, Ph.D., *Fed-Up: A Woman's Guide to Freedom from the Diet/Weight Prison* (New York: Carroll & Graf Publishers, 1993) p. 13.

especially professionals have trouble admitting that the risks of obesity have been exaggerated. A great many people who are statistically overweight are perfectly healthy; there is a wide range of healthy body sizes. As a result of that exaggeration, millions of people have spent billions of dollars trying fruitlessly to make themselves more healthy by going on diets. In doing so, they have neglected the serious health consequences, the physical and psychological cost, of dieting and yo-yoing weight.

But suppose it were effectively true that all fat is poison. Suppose we agreed that thin is always better and healthier and ensures a longer life than fat, the question would still remain: In whose life? Not in mine if, like most Americans, I'm getting fatter all the while I'm trying to diet and get exercise. And if I have to live my whole life struggling to be thin because I hate fat, if I make myself sick with dieting and weight watching, with the result that I keep on getting fatter, then my whole life is a failure, and I die early anyway. So why would I want to be thin? In fact, in fat, I am coming to look more like who I am, who is fat.

The shift in our relation to fat may be spurred by a growing awareness that the whole culture of dieting and rigid exercise is the root cause of the fat explosion. It may dawn on us collectively that telling people fat is bad for them and encouraging them to diet initiates physiological and psychological mechanisms that quickly result in our getting fatter. Obesity may be an iatric disease—that is, one caused by doctors, nutritionists, and health and beauty therapists. Unwittingly, of course, the diet system produces the disease that the system is charged with curing. Fat is decreed to be poison, but the antidote, diet and exercise, makes more fat, and a lot more money for the health-fitness-beauty industry. There is reason to think that if doctors stopped threatening people about their weight they would be thinner. Proving that is not easy, but maybe not impossible. The proposition would find instant verification if there were a shift in our attitudes toward fat. If we started to love it, we might stop getting fatter

In the meantime, we haven't. The National Health and Nutrition Examination Survey estimates that 58 million adult Americans are statistically overweight.* At the moment, Americans are the fattest people in the world. At least among industrialized nations. It is true, by comparison, that among Western Samoans, 76.8 percent of women are obese and are loved for their fat by Samoan men. But in North America, at any given moment, fully 40 percent of women (and 15 percent of men) are on weight-loss diets.† Only a third of women are statistically overweight, but 85 percent say they are preoccupied with losing fat.

It is probably incorrect to say, as have some, like the American Health Foundation, headed by Surgeon General Koop, that Americans have been gaining weight steadily. In fact, according to Robert J. Kuczmarski of the National Center for Health Statistics, who co-authored a recent study published in the *Journal of the American Medical Association,* the increase was relatively flat from 1960 to 1980. But from 1980 to 1991, at the height of the diet and fitness craze, American weight increased by 8 percent. He cited various reasons for the increase, including "the decrease in smok-

---

* *Life,* February 1995.
† *Toronto Star,* May 21, 1995.

ing, the increase in fast-food restaurants, the use of VCR's and jobs where people sit glued to computers."° It is amusing to speculate that Surgeon General Koop, who arguably has done more than anyone to suppress smoking, may be responsible for the increase in weight among all the ex-smokers his work has produced. The doctors' report makes no mention of the fact that during the same period, coinciding with the Reagan administration, the number of the poor has grown. Becoming poor in this country is synonymous with an increased likelihood of growing fat.

A lot of men and women I know—including myself—think about fat every day of their lives. I look in the mirror and register fat; I push against the sink and feel my paunch. I change clothing and notice, stand up and feel it bearing down, lie down and sink into the accommodating pillows of my fat couch. And I am not alone. Every sign says we are a people obsessed with fat, our own and others', in the can and on the shelf, in our veins and on the plate. Fat is everywhere around and within—the very ether in which many of us increasingly are living our lives. Our individual self-image, the image in the mirror we seek to project, and with it our sense of self-worth are shadowed by the negative values we assign to fat. Those values are inculcated in us while very young by the culture in which we grow up.

Dieting starts earlier and earlier; it has grown to be common among nine- and ten-year-old girls. Fortunes are being wagered on the search for a magic bullet with which science one day will deliver us the gift, in the form of a pill, of being thin. But until that

° *Los Angeles Times,* October 18, 1994.

moment, American behinds, seen on tourists and on television, are likely to remain the butt of jokes in every culture but our own.

There is abundant evidence to suggest that attempts to curb your appetite voluntarily encourage the body to make fat, incite the impulse to binge, and are the precipitating cause of many eating disorders. Only four people out of a hundred continue, after dieting, to keep their weight down: 76 percent of all dieters are fatter after three years than they were before they began, and 95 percent after five years. Eating disorders have recently been reported to be twice as widespread as had been thought, and the incidence is steadily rising. According to the *Times*, "the single most likely culprit for the rising rate of . . . eating disorders, experts say, is the spread of dieting."*

The moment one begins to deprive oneself, physically or psychologically, the body and the mind, faced with the specter of starvation, are programmed to find ingenious metabolic strategies for restoring the previous condition. They use food more efficiently and consume it more compulsively in order to make even more fat, which is more difficult to lose.

Some people actually lose weight when they stop dieting. But giving up diets may, in the end, be even harder for many people than restricting their food. To decide to stop dieting ends the illusion that you are in control of your weight. It may mean, as well, deciding to abandon the dream of ever being thin, all hope of one day looking the way you thought you wanted to look, rather than the way you are. It's easy, in our society, to love thin, but hard to

---

* *New York Times*, October 4, 1994.

achieve it. It's easy to be fat today, but hard to love it. Rather than working to get thin we should all be working to love fat. Not in order to become more obese, although that may happen, but because fat is what most of us are becoming anyway. But at the end of this century, loving fat is even harder than dieting.

What is to be done? What else is there to do? Diet books proliferate and evil doctors foist new drugs on desperate people. Nothing works for long. Young women, and some men, are increasingly anorexic and bulimic. Eating disorders, occasioned by the neurotic conflicts surrounding fat, undermine their youthful strength, their already shaky adolescent confidence. Thousands die of starvation, and the rest, sooner or later, get fat.

The answer this book proposes may not make you thin. It's not evident that it will make you any fatter than you will get if you keep on dieting. You might even get thinner, and you'd certainly stop a lot of the obsessing that surrounds all the anxiety about being fat. And that might cause you to eat more healthily, without the excesses to which dieting forces us. But, hey, there are no guarantees. No one can say, with absolute assurance, what you will let happen to yourself if you let yourself do it.

Believe me, it isn't easy—today, in our culture, with all the messages coming down to eat no fat, less fat, low or lite fat, to eat fat free. But this is a postmodern diet book. What it's proposing is something like an anti-diet. Try this for six weeks: EAT

FAT.

I know it sounds like just one more recommendation put in the form of an order you are supposed to obey, at the cost of your freedom. Like diet books that tell you to do this or don't do that. But

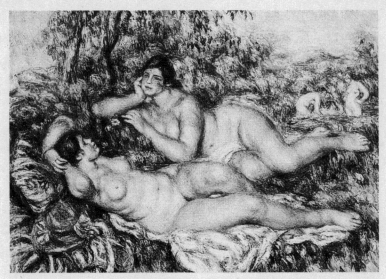

The Nymphs *by Renoir*

think a minute. What's the worst thing that could happen to you in six weeks, if you took this order seriously? Of course some people, with heart disease or diabetes, need to eliminate fat from their diet. But for the rest of us, more or less healthy, what's the worst that could happen?

Suppose you accepted obediently to follow the imperative, what exactly would you do? Go on a fat diet and eat only grease? Eat some sorts of fat but not others? Stuff your face with chocolate, more of the chocolate you may be sneaking enough of already? No fruits, vegetables, or grains—ever? Seriously, how long do you think you could let yourself eat grease, even if you had permission to eat all the grease you wanted? This is not a recommendation to eat grease, although it loves fat. It doesn't mean to eat fast, although fast can be fun.

How fat would you let yourself get if you were ordered, on pain of pain, never, for six weeks, to think of getting thin? Would you get fatter than we are all becoming already? Fatter than we Americans are getting by obsessively watching what we eat? If we stopped watching our weight, how much worse would it be?

If, dieting, we get fatter, it would seem to follow, like the night the day, that if you put the cover of *this* book on your fridge, you may get thin. Maybe you think I'm asking you to believe in some kind of reverse psychology. Or maybe this is what logicians call a pragmatic paradox. That's what they call, for example, an order that, if it were obeyed, would oblige you to do the opposite of what it commands.

Suppose, for example, I were to decree that you must

Stop reading this sentence!

In order to obey this order you have to disobey it, by reading and understanding it. By the same pragmatic logic, you might start to be thin if you were to grasp and follow the order, posted on your fridge, to EAT

FAT. But you'll see, there's a lot more to it than that, starting from the necessity, implicit in this title, to transvalue, to transform, and to reevaluate the value of fat.

In our culture, we've observed, fat is ugly. Fat is ugly on the inside and on the outside, on the shelf and in the freezer. Yesterday (April 26, 1995), the *New York Times* had a picture of a diet doctor holding a blob of yellow fat. It was artificially made, has the consistency of Jell-O, and sits on his desk to show fat clients the buttery horror under their skin. He displays it the way people who want you to stop smoking hold up an ashtray full of damp and dirty butts. Fat is repulsive and repugnant, he says to us, extending the blob toward the camera.

But there is fat and fat. If that fat had come from, say, the hips of Elizabeth Taylor, we might fall on our knees with gratitude for the pleasure it has given humanity. Suppose, God forbid, he was holding up a slab of the fat of Jessye Norman. We might not find it so ugly, we might honor it—some would worship this fat—that contributes in ways, known and unknown, to exuding the sweet power of the sound we love. What strength, both physical and psychological, does she derive from eating fat, from accumulating and storing and rarely losing any fat—on the contrary, from getting fatter all the time? Whatever it is, I honor that fat. The fat on James Beard represented the accumulation of a lifetime of the most persistent eating in the interest of bringing more of the pleasure of food to us all. I honor the sacrifices that that fat represents and envy the pleasure.

Imagine that what the doctor was holding up to the camera was not a greasy blob of yellow fat but a little suckling pig. If you look hard at the blob of fat Dr. Gullo is holding it does sort of look like a little pig with its fatty snout turned to the right. On the left it looks like a beautiful fetal child, secure in the fat that feeds it, which warms it and insulates it against the shocks inflicted by a cruel world and an abrupt or active mother. Or imagine that what the doctor is shoving at you is a lump of gold, of bright, sunny, beautiful gold. Like gold, fat is a treasure that those who fear starving store up, hoard, and find beautiful;

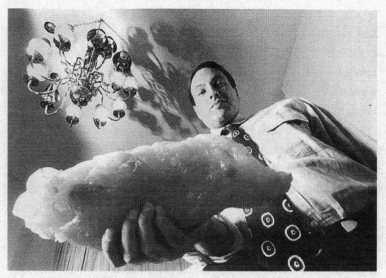

*Dr. Stephen Gullo with the five-pound yellow model of fat
he keeps on his desk*

they admire its abundance, love the security it provides, and relish the freedom it gives you in facing an uncertain future. Transvaluing fat into gold is the alchemical magic this book aims to effect.

But let's be clear. In our culture, fat is poison. Whether it's the fat on your hips or the fat in your food, being fat or eating fat is seen as a ticket to disease and early death: heart attacks or cancer, diabetes or stroke, to name a few. Obesity itself is widely considered to be a disease, both physical and psychiatric. Doctors everywhere discriminate against the fat, blaming and shaming them, holding them morally responsible, because of their fat, for any signs of ill health.

In our culture, fat is evil. Eating it or wearing it, feeding it or bearing it is a sign of some moral deficiency. Aesthetically, physically, and morally, fat is a badge of shame. A visible sign that in crucial areas of our life we have failed to be all we could be. An inescapable source of disappointment, of sadness and guilty self-contempt—of unrelenting shame.

To transvalue the value of fat in the present climate would take more than simple persuasion. Pasting the jacket of this book on your fridge can repeat the experience of reading this book, automatically, only because it's not a matter of persuading you of anything. There is no argument here I want to make or principle to teach. My fundamental purpose, the whole aim of this book, summed up in its title, is not to convince but to charm you. By that I don't only mean to please you or seduce you into accepting my arguments, in the common sense of charm; I mean as well something more literal, more concrete: this book aims to work like a charm, to cast a spell by conjuring a spirit—a compelling voice, repetitive, monotonous, as if from another world, that says over and over EAT

FAT.

This voice may sound absolutely alien, today, when fat is ugly poison and evil. It will be easy to show that at other times in history, and even today in other cultures, the message would be perfectly audible, well understood, fully acceptable, and enthusiastically embraced. But to persuade a reader today to love fat requires verbal powers more material than mere rhetoric. As far as I know there's only one way to make that kind of magic. It's what Nietzsche calls reinterpreting misery. It requires reversing the value of fat and thin.

Suppose, to take his example, you have a stinky little skinny stream, oozing through the middle of your otherwise stately garden. What do you do? You reinterpret its misery by erecting in its midst a lovely plaster nymph, at a strategic spot where the eye must pause, from whose charming urn the little stream now deliciously appears to flow. Nothing in the natural landscape has changed; only the meaning of the stream has altered, and its value has been reversed. Instead of being a sort of scar that marred the proportions of the garden, it appears now to be divinely fitted to be spilling precisely from the lip of that adorable urn, suspended on the hip of the superb little nymph, whose shape and size have been perfectly calculated by the cunning gardener. The misery of the actual stream has not been physically improved or altered in any way; only its context has changed. This is a piece of magic, because a sign, this statue, appears all by itself, like a fairy wand, to actually transform what's ugly into what's beautiful—what's thin into what's fat.

If this book succeeds, even a little, in changing the context of fat, then it might make magic, cast a spell however briefly, that allows the reader to grasp another perspective on fat. If this book succeeds if only for a moment in changing the value you give fat, then that might be a sign that all around us, at this very moment, the conditions are gathering for a general reversal. Changing your perspective on fat is the first step perhaps in a shift in fashion that once more will make fat beautiful.

For this is a postmodern diet book; it rejects the modern rejection of fat, the movement that began with twentieth-century industrialization and may be expiring in the age of virtual reality.

I locate the starting point of the thin look in *Les Demoiselles d'Avignon*. That famous painting by Picasso, in the Salon of 1909, caused a scandal; it was an early Cubist painting that instructed the viewer in the new perspective of Cubism, that showed the extent to which humans were being transformed by their machines. The streamlined forms of modern machines, the abstract geometries they enforce put limits on fat, set requirements and defined limits for the human component. Mechanical machines are prostheses—artificial limbs or senses—that extend the range and power of humans even while they transform the humans they serve. Postmodern machines are more abstract than mechanical—a neural extension, more like a computer than a sleek car. Modern machines are spare and efficient; postmodern machines are fat and all-consuming, excessive, luxurious, ill-defined.

Fat phobia is modern. The modern idea of thin beauty invented at the beginning of the century may at the end be giving way to a new idea of fat. Like a lot of postmodern architecture, fashion may be ready to cast back to an earlier era—for example, to a fin de siècle aesthetic that was fat and loved fat.

This book, or at least its cover—the reminder of this piece of magic, lets you have the experience of seeing fat from that other perspective, which changes everything. Those words, EAT

FAT, that round figure on the square page, on the jacket, are intended to be a kind of mandala—an image or sign that permits reflective meditation and transforms the participant in its labyrinths. In a way, the whole book is a reflection on the title, which both invites reflection and reflects the book as a whole—sums it up. Reading the title, you've already read everything you need to know for the book to work. In a way, you don't need to read any more. It's simply all there, in the title, EAT

FAT. Still, you have to read the book in order to understand what is already there—entirely contained in the title. It requires a whole book to say what the title says all by itself. But that's also why, once you've read the book, it's enough to see the title, pasted there on your fridge, for the whole effect of the book to be repeated, in order to reexperience the benefits that the book hopes to provide.

This is not a book of fat acceptance. Acceptance often means resignation, a reluctant willingness to accept what one cannot change but deep down would still love to. Fat acceptance demands tolerance from others but often continues to share the general hatred of fat in the form of self-hatred. If you have to accept your fat, then you probably still hate it, hate it as much as any lipophobic. The low self-esteem of most fat people implies that they have internalized the same general appreciation of fat that everyone else in society shares. And why shouldn't they, when they are daily the object of disdain and discrimination. Fat acceptance is a necessary step. Fat acceptance fights pernicious discrimination against fat. NAAFA, the National Association for the Advancement of Fat Acceptance, is the oldest and most important organization of Americans that defends the rights of fat people. But, insofar as the movement accepts what it can't change but would like to, it risks becoming a dead end, as much an obstacle as a prod to transformation. What differentiates this book from most fat acceptance books is that it doesn't wish to accept fat but to love it, and find it beautiful. At other times in history, in other cultures it wouldn't be hard to learn to love fat. And in fact, it's not hard to learn. Once you've decided you want to. That's the hard part.

The book tries to set out, in an orderly, systematic fashion, some of the meanings already contained in the title. But it doesn't expect or intend to exhaust them all.

It will consider:
the word *fat;*
the thing fat;
the idea or concept of it.

In order to transvalue the value of fat, we have to start by looking at the word. We have to observe and understand the way it's being used these days, repeatedly, obsessively, exuberantly, all around us. It is a word we see repeated hundreds of times every time we go to the supermarket. It must be one of the most abundantly reiterated words in print in the language, if you count all the times it appears on boxes on shelves.

There are not a lot of words in English, maybe not in any language, that can be repeated as often with as much pleasure as *fat*. I haven't finished counting all the times I'll use the word in this book, but I will. And you will be the judge of whether you can stand to hear the word another time. I'm still not tired of writing it.

The style of this introduction is supposed to be incantatory, to work like a mantra to change, if only briefly, the usual context of your thinking, through the suggestive power of verbal rhythms. This book is intended to be both mildly hypnotic and subtly, peculiarly erotic. Part of transvaluing the value of fat involves altering the way we hear the word, hearing differently in new or older ways, the word fat. I find as I write that I'm cultivating a fat style. I'm constantly trying to find ways to say f-f-fat, to say it over and over again because I believe in the necessity of that incantation. The whole style of this book is kind of bilious, ebullient alliteration, a sort of blustering stutter that sounds sometime like a buzz or hum of repeating words and echoing sounds that induce a low-grade alpha state, the condition of heightened receptivity. To start to EAT

FAT you

have to hear the word everywhere and hear it anew.

There's one point about the word *fat* that has to be made right away. Sometimes the word in English is a noun, sometimes an adjective—a thing or a quality of things. It's the adjectival sense, the attributes fat lends to things, that appears to belong to the oldest use of the word, where it means something like rich or fertile or bountiful. Since adjectives are often adverbial, the title EAT

FAT can be

understood, in a first sense, in an original sense, to mean not just to lap lipids but to eat fatly, abundantly, richly, and well. There was fat before there was civilization, but in civilization it has acquired significance in diverse ways across the ages and across the globe. In nature, fat is always "beautiful." I mean, positively appreciated, however dimly, by the animals who accumulate it. That it can become ugly in some cultures, changing the sign of its value from plus to minus, demonstrates the intertwining in fat of nature and culture.

When you go to the supermarket, try repeating the word, try saying it twice. Repeat it every time you see no-fat-less-fat-fat-free.

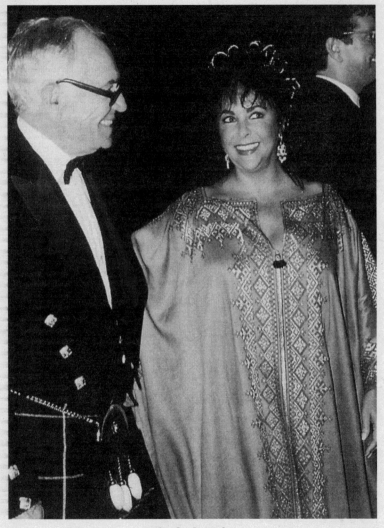

Elizabeth Taylor

Because repeating the fat word, adding the adjective to the noun, reveals the truth of what's in those containers. The repetition lets you hear what the no-fat-less-fat-fat-free label tries to hide. Bacon, for example, might be advertised as less-fat (fat), but it is fat just the same. No-fat (fat) is also fat; it's without fat but fatty nevertheless. In the unconscious, says Freud, there is no No! In the same way, there can be no no-fat the minute you have the fat (fat) word. It's always there superabundantly, always more and more fat fat.

Perhaps because fat is so many things. And because the word *fat* comprises so much, opens up to surround in its very idea so many diverse and finally universal realities. The Teutonic root for *fat* means to hold or contain, like a vessel, particularly a precious one containing baptismal water. Or like a tub. Everything that used to come in a tub or cask was good (oh! blessed), like fat or wine or beer. Everything tubby is fat. Fat denotes the well-supplied: fat purses, fat cheeses. Fat clay is pure; fat wine is fruity, full bodied; fat land yields abundant returns. A fat position is a desirable one, a fat kitchen is an affluent one, and a fat kingdom is where we live.

There must have been a time when everything that came in vats was good. Vats of things were what you desired above all to possess. Security against the Siberian winters of Dark Age Europe. Back then, all the good things that made life safe, bearable, and even intoxicating came in vats. Since fat came from vat, and vats contained fat, we assume that the word got its name by metonymy: what is contained, good yellow fat, gets its name from what surrounds and encloses it, its container, vat. It's true no doubt that fat can be stored in vats, against the future, but fat itself is a vat. Fat itself stores up energy in the form of fat molecules that can be released to be broken down as nourishment for body cells. Fat is the cellar of our body, where we keep our vats in fat.

At its root, vat is a verb that means to hold, to contain, to surround and enclose. It is related in German to the verb *fassen*, which means to grasp, and is very close in its meaning to the idea in German for "concept": in German a concept is *ein Begriff*, something that seizes hold, grasps, and comprehends many different things in the clutch of a single encompassing idea. You might say that the difference between *begriffen* and *fassen*, between grasping and containing, is between an active and a passive, a male and a female way of taking hold and containing: *grasp* (*begriffen*) is active, masculine seizing fast and hard; *fat* (*fassen*), like *vat*, is passive, embracing, enclosing—the enveloping hug that secures what cannot be easily gathered up and held. Fat has often, throughout history and until very recently, been thought to be feminine.

Fat like a vat, like a concept, surrounds and holds things together. Justice, for example, includes within its grasp a great many different sorts of things about which we feel secure in saying that they belong to the realm of what is just. The single concept, justice, like a great vat, contains many widely different forms and includes a vast number of examples of what is just. But the concept, like a vat, doesn't contain just any sort of things, it contains only the things that belong to it. In a tub or a vat, you put only things that belong together, like wine or fat. When you go to a vat you expect to find only the thing it contains. The same goes for a concept.

What vats of fat contain, it's fair to say, is sunshine. Fat stores the energy of the sun, accumulated and reserved in cells all up and down the food chain. Nuts have fat, as do larvae of insects; the fetus has fat, as does the coconut. All seeds and eggs and germs of things have plenty of little vatlike cells that store fat, which contains the energy the organism uses when external sources of food are unavailable.

A vat containing fat contains a container, because fat too contains, reserves, stores up. Taking a vat of fat as a concept, since it contains a container, is saying that it's the concept of the concept; it represents the idea of what an idea is and does. A vat of fat is the essential fatness that contains the very idea of fat. A vat holds fat, which holds—sunshine. Holding what holds, a vat of fat holds itself, like the idea of the idea. In other words, the concept of concept is like a vat of fat: it encloses what encloses—what surrounds, delimits and defines, reserves and stores up for future use—fat, concept. In a way, thinking about a vat of fat is like thinking about thinking in general.

Maybe that's why fat seems so important to me. It's got to be important, since it's one of the first and last things I think about every day of my life. Besides the word, besides the concept, there's, after all, the thing, fat, in concrete, material fact. I know a lot of people like me, particularly women, but a lot of men, too, who confront the thing, fat, every day. Most of us, when we look in the mirror at night and in the morning don't look admiringly at the beauty of our bodies, we look at our bodies and see fat. In a mostly negative way fat is the thing that reminds many of us every day that we have a body. It's amazing how a glance in the mirror or a moment on the scale can instantly lower or raise the measure of our self-esteem. Fat is a thing that has a natural existence, inside and outside me. Even when it belongs to me it's something I'd rather like to lose. My fat is part of me—not. It is heterogeneous to who I am, not me at all but what I'd like to lose—yet all too well homogenized. Fat is a thing that has a nature and a history; it's organic but it's full of meaning, acquiring many different meanings at different times in history, and across cultures. When I look in the mirror and I see the thing fat, I am not seeing it through the eyes of a man, say, in the seventeenth century, standing before a glass and admiring his stout and florid embonpoint. Nor are mine the eyes of a prosperous German in 1965, looking pridefully on fat as irrefutable proof of his newly great prosperity, an index of his moral substance and a tool for imposing, even intimidating, in social space.

What I see when I look at fat is a thing both physical and cultural, both a measurable mass of cellular mush and a whole image of myself in relation to some idea I have of my own beauty. When I look at the glistening bar of butter on the plate, like the animal I am I recognize its value and love its qualities and anticipate its sensual pleasures. I also see it through the eyes of the slight taboo that causes me to have an instantaneous shiver of displeasure, of mild guilt at the thought of so much fat, at the price of the fat on my hips and in my arteries. The thing before me, the fat on my pot or on my lips, is more than a mere substance, whose role and function, whose value and use can be decided by experts, medical, nutritional, or otherwise.

The place of fat in our lives has a long history, before history even began. It was placed at the center of human thought, conscious and unconscious, for millennia before civilization acculturated it, doubled it, made it fat fat: a substance and an attribute that intersect the realms of biology and language.

Maybe we are so obsessed with fat because each pound we add is like a measurable sign of growing old. Growing old is growing fat. To be thin is to be young, and the prestige of the young in our culture needs no commentary. Somehow it's more consoling to think that growing fatter as we age is a mere lapse of control, attributable to our character, capable of being disciplined, halted, and reversed. We think we can control our fat, because we can't control our aging.

Suppose you were a middle-aged man like me, watching with inexorable necessity the growing accumulation of fat around your stomach. You've been sufficiently motivated to exercise seriously most of your life, but for some time you haven't been any thinner than what you are now. Which is fat. Maybe it's your breakfast. I can't stop returning to breakfast.

I would guess that fifty percent of the fat that I bear comes from those breakfasts. I have crumbly bacon and two fresh eggs over easy, biscuits and grits when I'm here in the South, fresh Florida orange juice, and double espressos. But some memorable breakfasts I have eaten in the early hours of a bitter cold morning in Ithaca, New York, when an ice-sharp wind coming off the lake cuts through layers of clothes like a laser from hell. Finding yourself on such a morning in the warmth of the Ithaca diner is a small solace, but an important one. At that moment when you need every kind of human warmth your solitude doesn't normally provide, at that moment God is in the grill, in the grease, in the slight intoxication that illuminates the congregation gathered on such an early morning shift in the glimmer of palest dawn. In the grill is the grease that feeds the diner—the focus of all our prayers that morning, the gift of love and the bond of community anonymously forged in diners, in every roadside stand in America. Perfumed with the faint smell of bacon grease, eggs frying in hot butter on the grill hiss and pop, all white and papal gold, afloat in the sizzling film of fat. I watch the cook in deep devotion at the grill, a sweet smile on her face; she doesn't look, but she's glad to see me; she offers me breakfast straight, before any waitress intervenes. She slips me an extra piece of toast, heavily buttered, I really don't need, but it's the wafer of communion with her I need. I eat it all, because she loves me. Because with the wind howling and the snow sweeping through barely plowed streets, that fat is a kiss, between her and me. It represents the sun, the sun absent from this frigid world, the sun that grows grass that feeds pigs that feed me bacon—crispy, melting, satiny sunshine, its beigy brown warmth dissolving beneath my tongue, singing a song of greasy sweetness that cheers the sun up. Warm skies and easy living are in my bacon and in the thick amalgam of yellow yolk and melting meat that starts my day with a little vat of fat. On my plate. In my mouth. It's the fat that gets me going in the morning, and the coffee. It gets me going happily, gaily even, up the hill to the darkened offices where I work.

But even here, in Florida, in the midst of the hottest summer in human history, there have been mornings when I've driven for an hour trying to find a breakfast place that's open, when I didn't have something in the fridge. I don't eat bacon and eggs every morning, no more than three or four times a week. Only when I need more fat.

Today, 49 percent of American women wear size 14 or larger, according to the National Panel Data Group, a New York research firm. Nearly 32 percent wear size 16 or larger. And this segment spent $12 billion on clothing last year. The plus-size industry generally caters to sizes 14W to 28, but some stores stock sizes 30 to 32.°

You speak to someone in the garment industry, they'll tell you that she's a tough customer, the plus-size-and-larger consumer of women's clothes. Under the weight of a social stigma, she hates to shop, she buys from catalogues, she doesn't rush out to get the latest thing that she absolutely has to have. For the garment business, there are no quick profits in plus sizes—miracles of retailing when suddenly something explosively takes off and everyone has to have it—a sleeveless black dress. Nevertheless, the market for plus-size clothes has shown slow but strongly consistent growth—as more and more fat women choose to buy better clothes and as we all get increasingly fat.

From the standpoint of the garment merchant, the fat customer is a reluctant shopper, and a tight one. She's very price sensitive, very conscious of expense. Selling plus sizes is a contrarian business, because it defies common sense. Thin people think fat shoppers want to hide their fat beneath discreet and unobtrusive clothing, the better to disguise what they loathe having to display to a stigmatizing world. On the contrary, and in fact, most of the fat shoppers seem to want large prints and bright colors, all the glitz and glop and flashing tchotchkes you can drip on a dress or pile on a mound of flesh. She hides behind the act of making herself highly visible; she conceals her body beneath the glamour of flashy accessories, bright colors, and big prints that command the eyes of others to look. Afraid that her fat body may provoke a scandal, she scan-

° *Atlanta Journal and Constitution,* May 28, 1995.

dalizes with the boldness of her clothes and accessories; she antici-pates the effect of her fat and seeks to defuse it by seeming to choose to want to provoke it. The more it seems she ought to want to conceal her fat, the more she flaunts it, as if to take control of the response she excites in others.

A man, I'm not supposed to be as preoccupied about fat as women. Women are obliged to consider thin as a precondition for success. A man of course doesn't feel the same pressure, but the pressure is there and it's internalized. Not only does the world mostly hate his fat, he hates it most himself.

It might seem easier if this book aimed to change our per-spective on fat by changing the value of thin. Lean, traditionally, is mean; seven lean cows in Joseph's dream mean seven years of famine for the pharaoh; fat cows promise seven years of abundant plenty. Hence, fat Falstaff's defense of fat in Shakespeare's *Henry IV: Part I:* "If to be fat is to be hated, then pharaoh's lean kine (cows) are to be loved." Who could love a skinny cow? Who could prefer thin if thin is starvation? Only an anorexic. Or us. Most of the models whose beauty obsesses the media at this moment have thin, emaciated arms. The models are probably starving. For most of us, to be as thin as you'd have to be to look thin or to correspond to what is called your ideal weight, at this moment of history you would have to starve, drink coffee, and smoke cigarettes, which at least a third of adults and most models are doing.

Whereas anorexic men are increasingly being diagnosed and described, the preponderance of eating disorders is found in women. Many of those women are obeying their parents' explicit orders or implicit wishes by a form of ironic revolt: defying their wishes, they fulfill them beyond their wildest dreams—to the last literal letter of the law. So you want me to be thin, I'll show you thin. The anorexic is a good girl, who does exactly what her parents wish, but in spades—to the death.

It's hard to hate thin at a moment when most American women are more or less on diets at any given time; famine has little power to move them. They are already trying to starve themselves. Most of them are starving, all too voluntarily, when they aren't busy gaining weight. It has been demonstrated that some radical diets provide the same level of nourishment, less than 900 calories, as that of inmate diets in Buchenwald. But in the eyes of many, the starving at Buchenwald must have their own peculiar beauty. Some of the commentators recently describing the victims in Somalia couldn't help but remark on the elegance of their elongated, fatless forms— skeletons, they nevertheless embodied (or disembodied) a certain current ideal of beauty, just as starving supermodels have become our culture's most glamorous icons.

All signs point to the fact that the ideal of beauty, as portrayed in the media and reflected in taste, has been growing steadily, alarmingly skinnier:

> From 1959 to 1978, the weights of women lounging in *Playboy* centrefolds dropped from 91 per cent of the age-height-adjusted average of all women to 84 per cent. At the same time, Miss America contestants also got smaller. Only 5 per cent of female bodies fit the misguided social ideal. Many of the remaining 95 per cent are unnecessarily unhappy, believing themselves condemned to life in a hellish body prison.°

° *Toronto Star,* May 21, 1995.

It is one of the assumptions of this book that fat is feminine and hence beautiful. But it's important to distinguish fat's beauty from the misguided idea or perverse ideal of what we normally think of as feminine beauty. That idea belongs to what Naomi Wolf calls the "beauty myth."* It is invented, manufactured, sustained, and promoted by a vast industrial, ideological system, in order to obscure the reality of our bodies. The myth is designed to oppress and exploit us all, but mostly women, with the notion that we can never be too thin. Since Twiggy, the look of anorexia has been chic. At the ballet the illusion of movement and grace is enhanced by the thinness of limbs that dancers, more and more, have begun to cultivate. Those women who have to look like internees in concentration camps or like citizens of a city under siege must starve themselves. The price they pay for a certain kind of feminine beauty is infertility.

Fat may be bad for some things, but there's lots of evidence that a fair amount of it is good for bearing children. There's no doubt that women who starve themselves eventually cease to menstruate and that fat may be necessary, particularly in uncertain times, to protect the growing fetus from any interruption of nourishment suffered by the scavenging adult. It's one of the constant puzzlements this book seeks to understand. Given all the genetic, all the biological reasons that must contribute to our being fat, and that may even explain why we are getting fatter, it seems, on the surface, strange that our current ideal of beauty, the anorexically thin, is so at odds with our biological requirements. It may be the paradox of style. For most of history, fat was a beneficent, produc-

* Naomi Wolf, *The Beauty Myth: How Images of Beauty Are Used Against Women* (New York: Doubleday, 1992).

tive, life-sustaining substance—a guarantee against the permanent dangers of scarcity, a spur to female fertility, an insulation against the cold winds that blow into primitive houses, a sign of abundance, a token of good cheer. Fat has throughout most of history been infinitely preferred to thin. So modern style decrees that thin is in.

In Tonga today, women are fattened for marriage, and thin is sickly. That was already true in the middle of the nineteenth century, when people's fears were tubercular, and stout meant hale and hearty. Among certain gay men in New York today, plumpness is taken, no doubt misleadingly, as a positive sign of health. But maybe, in fact, a lot of gay guys are having sex less and eating more, the next best thing to sex. The value of fat has been so devalued that it takes a minor miracle, a trick or sleight of hand, a little epiphany, in order to glimpse an alternative: a world in which fat is affirmed and appreciated and loved—in which fat in all its forms is once again blessed—fair fat, fine fat, fresh and fluffy fat fabulously fit.

Believe me, it isn't easy to transvalue fat. Most people hate it— on other people and on themselves, in the supermarket or at the gym. Much has been written in the last ten years or so demonstrating the forms and origins of fat phobia (which is not at all the same thing as phat fobia, as we will see). The *Journal of Social and Clinical Psychology* published research that showed that it takes just three minutes for women, albeit American women, to be traumatized by pictures of supermodels. Nearly seven out of ten end up suffering from "Barbie syndrome"—feelings of depression, stress, guilt, and shame.* Just as Barbie proportions are unreal, the shape of those emaciated models is genetically, realistically beyond the

* *London Sunday Telegraph,* January 8, 1995.

reach of nearly all the women who are ashamed by comparison. This is tragic—the internalization by these women of an ideal of beauty at such an impossible, unhealthy distance from their own bodies. It understandably stirs the rage of those like Naomi Wolf who see the beauty myth as an iron maiden with which a male-dominated society tries to constrain and hobble women, to undermine their confidence and strength at the moment they are everywhere acceding to power.

Look closely at zines like *Top Model,* at the anatomy of some supermodels, such as Claudia Schiffer and Linda Evangelista, whose bodies conform to no ideal of feminine beauty ever observed in history, with the exception of some late Gothic paintings of ethereal, self-abnegating saints. The bodies of those top models betray, often unexpectedly, the traces of starvation, of purging, of the substances they ingest in order to avoid ingesting food. How fat could a top model get before she stopped being top?

Today, it's hard even to remember when fat was loved, although it wasn't all that long ago. Nineteenth-century pornography, like what you see on old postcards, depicts mostly women who are fat. There's a famous picture taken by Brassaï in La Lune Bleue, a celebrated bordello in Paris in the twenties. An eager, handsome, smiling young man is just coming in, taking off his coat before he ever gets through the door. He's greeted by the Madam, chicly dressed and very fat. Surrounding her are three women of the house, completely naked except for their high heels. Two of them are enormous, by our standards, shapely but very fat, with small breasts and large hips and great bellies. The most astonishing thing in the photo is the smile of wicked anticipation on the face of the young, handsome, probably rich young man, as he contemplates the pleasure he will pay for with these obese, lascivious, expensive women. One cannot imagine any adolescent today fantasizing an erotic adventure in a house with women who look monstrous, terrifying, impotent-making women to most American males. In her long history the goddess Venus has mostly been fat. But these days, it's not often we are turned on by fat, and those who are, are viewed with suspicion. Fat has become an obscenity, something that ought to but cannot be hidden well, that exhibits itself only as something deforming, ugly, disruptive of your sense of self, like a scarlet letter, the oleaginous yellow of *F*. In Ireland a good stout girl was traditionally desired by men, who had reason to respect the strength and resistance of women we would consider obese.

Take a good look at Edna Ann Evangelista Rivera, whose picture is one of those collected in *Women En Large*.* Is she beautiful, though fat? Is she desirable, I mean hot? Maybe it's just the way she's propped on the umbrella, as on a sword, and, a fetishist, I fall for phallic mothers. Maybe it's the alluring texture of her skin against the fierce lifeless surface of the lava rock. Or the way her eyes smolder with curiosity and suspicion, her right foot turned as if she's about to run away, her left firmly planted where she stands. Your eye keeps coming back to those eyes, like two camera lenses peering at you from the top of a tripod, like the one formed by her legs and the umbrella. Fat people, without self-esteem, offer themselves up passively to be viewed, as if in a spectacle—the fat lady, the fat man. Not Edna Rivera. She knows she's beautiful. But if you asked any woman

---

* Laurie Toby Edison and Debbie Notkin, *Women En Large: Images of Fat Nudes* (San Francisco: Books in Focus, 1994).

you know if she would like to have a body like hers, what would she say? If you asked her if she would like to be as fat as Edna, you pretty much know how she'd answer. It's true of course that roughly 50 percent of Hispanic-American women, slightly less than African-American women, are clinically obese. That genetic fact may also be linked to the great poverty in those groups; in America, in the nineties, there is a strict correlation between your socioeconomic class and your chances of being fat. The richer you are, the more likely you will be thin. But in Hispanic- and African-American cultures, fat is assigned a different value, one that in America often coexists with, even while it contradicts, the dominant negative one.

In Britain, two women called Stephanie and Fay run Positive Plus Sizes (PPS), which was started in order to bring together Afro-Caribbean and other black women whose cultures generally assume that the fatter you are, the healthier you are. The group practices resistance to advertising and to social pressures on such women to conform to the white anorexic idea of beauty. Classes run by Stephanie and Fay, who are both winners of the Big and Beautiful contest, seek to bolster the confidence of black women and raise their self-esteem.

Maybe they don't really need it. A University of Arizona survey found that young black girls have an infinitely more positive image of themselves than white adolescents. In a survey of 250 teenagers, 90 percent of white girls were dissatisfied with their bodies, compared to 70 percent of blacks, who said they were satisfied with their bodies and not interested in dieting. The white girls' emphasis was on thinness, while the black girls spoke about shapeliness.

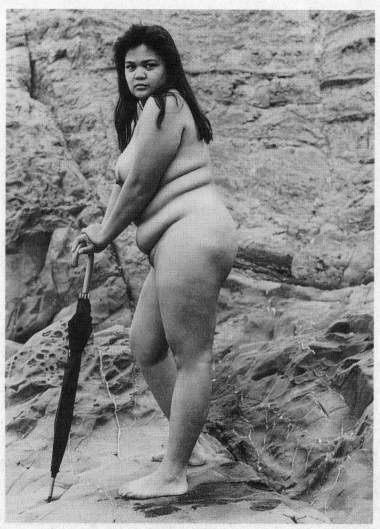

Edna Rivera

Shapeliness rather than fat may be the crucial factor determining sexual desirability; the smaller the waist in relation to the hip, the more desirable a woman is seen to be. Professor Devendra Singh at the University of Texas believes that this may be the most powerful sexual trigger of all, and what strengthens her theory is the fact that this ratio has recently been recognized as a key indicator of health.*

No other animal has a waist; according to Dr. Singh, once humans stood up, they needed bigger buttocks, to support an upper body supported now only by two legs. Since we are human, we can have bubble butts. In a series of experiments, Dr. Singh found that men had a clear reaction to different waist-hip ratios. In a survey of 106 men aged 18 to 22, the favorite was a female of average weight with the classic hourglass figure. Not only were such women rated as young, sexy, and healthy, they were also seen as ideal for childbearing. In Dr. Singh's other surveys, men of all ages agreed with these findings, bearing out her theory of the waist-hip ratio. Perhaps it is this ratio that explains fashion's seeming regression to uplift bras and, lately, corsets. Claudia Schiffer, the German top model, is one of the few beings in the world who manages simultaneously to be emaciated and curvy; the other of course is Barbie, whose proportions if realized in a human would require removal of the stomach and most of the reproductive organs.

But the illusion persists, and despite the growing preponderance of fat, in our culture it remains an ugly word, a wretched thing, an unflattering idea. Face it, fat is foolish, fat is funny, fat is no fun. It takes some measure of imagination to be fatiloquent, which

---

* *Dublin Irish Times*, November 10, 1994.

means prophetic, and imagine a day when the value of fat may be radically transformed in the world. It takes some memory to remember when fat was fine. It would take a minor miracle to glimpse, even briefly, the possibilities of another world, in which we loved fat—all things fat and good. Hillel Schwartz has demonstrated the necessity and sketched the outlines of such a world. In a chapter entitled "A Fat Society: A Utopia," he writes, "If the table could be turned, if this were a fat society, a society that admired and rewarded fatness—a society that has never existed in this country, for both sexes at the same time—things would be very much different and very much better."*

Fair fat, fine fat can only be conjured up, in the time of a flash—with the wave of a wand. You get it or you don't. Only if you can catch a glimpse, open a window on a new vista, can you respond, again and again, to the magic in the title, every time you read EAT

FAT.

It is important, as a first step into the mandala, that you hear this title as a reply to all the orders coming down to eat thin. They are coming down on every side. All around we are being urged to eat no fat, less fat, fat-free foods, we are driven to cut fat, exhorted to move our fat, and warned to lose it because of our health. Being fat, we are the objects of threats and judgments, often implicit, that concern our character and shape our future. Fat, we are held up for ridicule by children, treated to the ritual scolding of parents,

---

* Hillel Schwartz, *Never Satisfied: A Cultural History of Diets, Fantasies, and Fat* (New York: Free Press, 1986), p. 324.

and delivered over to widespread contempt and derision. Fat, we secretly amuse our friends—if they are thinner than we are. Assuming we have any thinner friends. The fatter we get, the more liable we are to be discriminated against for our fat—erotically, professionally, civicly. Some of us are tragically thin, out of fear of fat. And even those of us who, being fat, lose weight and appear thin are still in our mind's eye the same old fatty we've always been.

Above all, in our culture being fat means you get no love, because you deserve no love. Being fat, and therefore failing to be the person you ought to be, probably could be, certainly *will* be one day (dammit), you have no right to receive any love—if you love yourself so little as to be fat. That's the message the world conveys and that you get every day from your mirror, as we all get fatter and fatter. Look in the mirror and see the expanse of your gut, the roll on your hip, and tell me you don't feel ashamed. You've let yourself go, and look at you. In the mirror, in your mind's eye, you have fallen short, by getting fat, of the ideal that alone could bring you satisfaction, pleasure, and, in all likelihood, wealth.

Most of us feel more or less of the time that we don't deserve to be loved, because of some vice or habit, some excess to which we are prone. But normally the source of our shame is hidden from immediate view, unobserved, if often suspected, by those around us. The nightmare of being fat is that your vice is visible, assuming of course, which should by no means be granted, that people who are fat are out of control.

Being fat, the source of your shame, the nature of your vice, is visible to everyone, even if overeating is not your vice. The world, seeing your fat, thinks it's justified in drawing conclusions about what it thinks it knows you've been doing or haven't been doing—eating or exercise. And the world barely takes the trouble to hide from you that it sees you are shamefully fat. Your fat is the mirror in which you are seen and see yourself being seen by others. Fat, in our culture, is obscene, in the sense that obscenity means making visible more than ought to appear. That's part of what makes it obscene. Being fat is making a spectacle of yourself like the fat little girl in Margaret Atwood's novel:

> The problem was fairly simple: in the short, pink skirt, with my waist, arms and legs exposed, I was grotesque. I am reconstructing this from the point of view of an adult, an anxious prudish adult like my mother or Miss Flegg; but with my jiggly thighs and the bulges of fat where breasts would later be and my plump upper arms and floppy waist, I must have looked obscene, senile almost, indecent; it must have been like watching a decaying stripper.[*]

Fat people, like the very old, ought not to be exposed to view; they are obscene when they are seen in public, like "a decaying stripper"—someone whose flesh ought to be veiled, not displayed. Just to look at them is to see too much. And yet, the indecency of the little girl's fat, hideously sexual before any sexual development has occurred, touches something deep in us, some form of the grotesque that needs to be explored.

[*] Margaret Atwood, *Lady Oracle* (Toronto: McClelland-Bantam, Inc., 1977), p. 42.

What is a fatty? That is a question it will be one of the aims of this book to answer. But we can say, in a preliminary way, that a fatty is a person who eats fat, not thin—with no intention to watch what he eats in order to be less fat. Take, for example, the nameless hero—I guess you could call him the hero—of Raymond Carver's little story called "Fat,"* He has a strange way of speaking, when he orders his dinner, and makes a little puffing sound every so often:

> I think we will begin with a Caesar salad, he says. And then a bowl of soup with some extra bread and butter, if you please. The lamb chops, I believe, he says. And baked potato with sour cream. We'll see about dessert later.

Seeing about dessert later doesn't mean weight watching, as if the fatty might actually pass up dessert. It just means that dessert is not exactly part of the meal; it's what you eat after you've had your dinner, when you can't eat any more. That's when you find room to eat more than you can eat—and that's dessert.

This guy is so fat that when the narrator of the story, who happens to be his waitress, comes out of the kitchen, she bumps into Margot, the other waitress: "Margot—I've told you about Margot? The one who chases Rudy? Margot says to me, Who's your fat friend? He's really a fatty."† Carver knows that we know that there

---

* Raymond Carver, "Fat," in *Will You Please Be Quiet, Please?* (New York: McGraw-Hill Company, 1978).
† Ibid., p. 2.

is some kind of sexual mystery surrounding people that he calls tubbies. You can't stop looking, talking about them, behind their backs. There's something sexy about a fatty, about excess with an edge of violence exciting anxiety, eliciting commentary and fascinated attention.

Consider the main character of Maupassant's first short story "Boule de suif," the nickname of a fat whore—a beautiful, touching, courageous, generous butterball. Nameless, with only a nickname in the story, she is a ball of the finest fat.

> The woman next to him, one of those described as of easy virtue, was locally famous for her tremendous rotundity which had earned her the nickname of Butterball (*Boule de suif*). Short, all curves, with flesh bulging from every part of her, with each finger like three fat little sausages strung together at the joints, with a tight and shiny skin and an immense bosom that overflowed from her dress—she was nevertheless extremely appetizing and very much in demand, so delightful was her freshness to the eye. Her face was like a red apple, like a peony bud about to bloom, and in the middle of it, there opened two superb dark eyes shaded by long thick eyelashes and, below them, a charming mouth, small and moist—a mouth made for kisses and furnished with small gleaming teeth. She also had a reputation for many other priceless qualities.*

* Guy de Maupassant, *"Boule de suif" and Selected Stories* (New York: Signet, 1964), p. 172.

In French, *boule de suif* doesn't refer at all to butter, but to cooking fat, to the greasy tallow used for candles, to the fat of geese and chickens or of a hare pâté. "It was one of those dishes with a china hare on its lid to indicate that inside a hare in the form of *pâté* was buried under a succulent assortment of charcuterie with white rivers of lard running through the brown flesh of the game mixed with other fine meats [201]" She herself, Boule de suif, is a vast *pâté*, running with rivers of lard, containing buried in its luscious grease the sweetest meats and the most surprising qualities beneath its charming exterior. This Butterball is a whole banquet in herself, an endless source of pleasure and good tastes, promising ever more delicate and delicious, more priceless pleasures within the curves of bulging flesh.

Peeking through a keyhole into Butterball's bedroom, one of the characters is aroused by the unexpected sight of her delicious rotundity, barely concealed beneath the delicate fabric of her frilly nightie. He caught sight of Butterball "looking more curvaceous than ever in a blue cashmere negligee with white lace trimmings."[*] The clinging blue cashmere accentuates her curves and frames in azure the shiny sleekness of the delicious flesh, peeking out of the lacy edges of her robe at the peeking voyeur behind the door. He is awed by the power of such abundantly beautiful flesh to arouse appetite and stir our deepest hunger.

Maupassant may have been one of those men who loved fat girls, like Rubens or Renoir. But these days such tastes can get you in trouble. Here's Jimmy Breslin writing, quoting Eva Lederman,

[*] Ibid., p. 184.

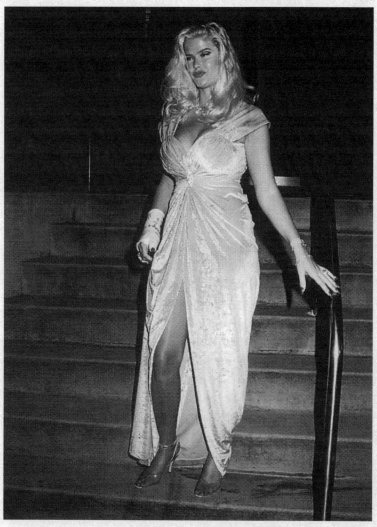

Anna Nicole Smith

head of a human rights group, Fight for Women: " 'Chubby chasers are a threat to women because they go after those most susceptible, those with a weight problem. You have to make these women understand that these men are vicious and sick. Whenever we talk about chubby chasers, the first remarks you hear from women are, "I haven't noticed one of them around yet. Where are they?" Or, "Show me where they are." But the charming remarks fade as they hear of the damage caused by these hideous men.' "*

Loving fat is defined in this view not only as an eccentric choice, like that of those who love only very thin people, but it is seen as perverse. It displays an interest in a fat woman as if she were nothing but her lard, instead of the richly complicated human being she is. The attraction of the chubby chaser to fat is judged in this perspective to be a pathological perversion, a hideous compulsion, a sickness that is also particularly vicious—as if these chasers were both helpless to resist loving fat and were wicked for doing it, as if they had both a choice and no choice to love a woman for her fat. A man who loves a fat woman, in this view, is supposed to love the thin person she is inside, the true self who hates her own fat as much as you do. Except you don't hate it. You love her fat, for what it fatly is. One woman, says Breslin, was followed by a man who persistently asked her out to lunch. "Then she found out he was a 'chubby chaser.' She was angry and frustrated. It reinforced her dream of having a man who wants her in spite of her build." She wants him to love her in spite of her fat or her size, not because of it—as if she were not in any way her fat. It is one of the premises of this book

* *New York Newsday,* November 13, 1994.

that your fat is not what you have but who you are. That doesn't mean you can't change who you are and get thin, but it probably requires that you undergo a kind of conversion, a transformation in the axioms with which you understand your experience.

Systematic surveys have confirmed that obese women generally prefer thin men and take the same disdainful attitude toward fat as most people do. In their eyes, as in those of most people, the chubby chaser is a menace, not a mensch; a real man doesn't love fat. FAs, as they call themselves, fat admirers, take a starkly different view. They consider themselves nothing more than a range of ordinary people: thin, average, or somewhat overweight guys who prefer fat women.

And FAs have problems finding fat women who will allow themselves to be loved for who they are, namely fat. Most fat women are consumed by shame and self-hatred. "Female fat admirers find fat men with relative ease; it's harder for male FAs to find fat women with self-esteem," said Sally Smith, executive director of the 4,000-member National Association to Advance Fat Acceptance. That's why half the 1,400 men who belong to the organization are thin guys looking for fat women, she said. "Many fat women prefer thin men, it's true," Smith said. "All our lives, fat women are told we can't expect to attract what society says is attractive—thin men." And it's not unusual to find clinically obese women (defined as people 25 percent over their ideal weight) who've never dated anyone but thin guys. Fat admirers live hard lives, said Ruby Greenwald of Albany-based *Dimensions* magazine, a publication for FAs that estimates that 10 percent of all men are attracted to fat women.[*]

[*] *New York Newsday*, August 9, 1993.

NAAFA has a Date and Personals service that helps chubby chasers. "It is a dating program designed especially for fat people and for those who prefer the fuller figure, and for those who have no weight preference." It's not exactly clear why someone with no preference would join a dating club with those who prefer the "fuller figure"—fat fat. The NAAFA dating brochure explains the rationale of the service: "You don't have to worry about being matched up with someone who fits your personality but hates fat." But the thin partner always has a delicate problem; he or she can neither hate fat nor love it for its own sake, in order to be allowed to give love, without prejudice or perversion, to a fatty. You can understand the dilemma of thin men: They are looking for fat women with self-esteem, who love themselves fat; conversely, their women are seeking men who love them despite their being fat. In a fat utopia, at that moment when fat women accept and love their fat, when thin men find fat women with self-respect and self-love, then the fat-loving thin and the self-loving fat will make a couple made in heaven.

One reporter at a NAAFA convention interviewed a clean-cut doctor, thirty-two, who wouldn't give his name, lest he alarm his patients, but who confesses that fat women were once his "principal sexual interest." He was at the meeting to see if he had kicked the habit. "They were more lascivious," he muses, speculating as to the root of his old fetish. "They could keep going. And it's nicer to touch them, more corners to explore. And you can't be dominated by someone really thin, can you?" With a cheeky laugh, he adds, "Size does count, you see."*

---

* *Washington Post*, April 28, 1993.

But what is there to say of those fat men who love other fat men? At Bulk in London, big guys can hang out with other fatties and feel comfortably unthreatened by the usual hostility.[*] But then, Bulk is nothing like the standard gay club. "Bulk is, as short, chubby host Bobby Pickering says, 'for fat boys, big dykes and their admirers—a distinct minority with a distinct subculture.' "[†] Fat men and males who love fat males are a distinct minority. Being gay and fat for many growing up makes a painful combination. The Bulk, like the subculture itself, is both a refuge and place of self-assertion, a niche boutique for entrepreneurs and an environment for personal liberation.

It's not at all the same subculture as that of *Fat Girls,* fat lesbian women, whose zine, by that name, is one of the sources I have most thoroughly mined in order to understand the beauty of fat.

These days, being fat is often a way of opting out of sexual life. For many that is its chief utility. For lesbians, it is a way of signaling that they don't seek the attention of men. At the same time it can become itself a source of a whole other erotic life, between women, in which the value of fat is transformed.

It is equally possible to show that fat is always associated with bigness and bigness is associated normally with males. In Western species of humanoid, the male is consistently larger than the female, often markedly so, as in Scandinavia, while among the Chinese the difference in the size of men and women is insignificant. In the West, we have always given a preference to bigness over

[*] *Irish Times,* November 10, 1994.
[†] *Independent,* August 4, 1994.

smallness. No one has ever had the thought that his penis wasn't small enough. Where women are concerned, it's quite clear: growing fat in our culture means becoming more male.

Pat Califia has an amazing story called "Big Girls." One of the heroes is an enormously big, fat bull dyke called Kat.

> Kat liked fine presentable women with good legs and pretty faces. When she went out to dinner with them or took them shopping, they made an obvious couple and a striking one. She would look impassively at the men who noticed her partner and feel grim satisfaction when they dropped their eyes and took their prick energy elsewhere. Being big had its advantages.[*]

So a woman who gets very fat grows into a butch; adding fat tends to masculinize her, while it feminizes men. The big butch girls in Pat Califia's story are aware of the stereotype that implies that all big women can repair washing machines or change spark plugs. Frequently, that stereotype corresponds to the reality that lets fat women assume roles normally reserved to men, by virtue of the strength they acquire from bearing fat, and from imposing their bulk on the space around.

It's not surprising that fat works more generously for men. You've probably seen the posters of a certain Flabio, aka Michael Glover, who is 6 feet 6 inches tall, weighs just under 400 pounds, and vaguely, fatly, resembles the buffed male model called Fabio.

---

[*] Pat Califia, "Big Girls," in *Melting Point* (Boston: Alyson Publications, 1993), p. 15.

"They put out a casting call for a guy 100 to 200 pounds over-weight who would pose at the beach in bathing trunks," Glover said. "My agent answered it for me, and out of 75 guys, I got the job. More people look like Flabio than Fabio, and I'm trying to bring out that big is normal, that it's OK to be big."*

He named big-guy actors John Goodman and the late John Candy as role models. In ninth grade he was 6'2" and weighed 220 pounds. A lot of people who are big and fat have been that way since they were born. Their whole life they have been prematurely big, like the girl who at ten has reached her mother's ideal weight. Big gives you access to a premature adulthood. If you're as big as an adult, you get treated like more of one, and at some point very early on you begin to appear to be forty-two years old, which is the age most fat people appear to be regardless of their age. Flabio is also in some way the truth of Fabio—the Flabio waiting to get out. Those puffed-up pec-torals, larger than life, have a way of suggesting their eventual trans-formation from muscle into flabby fat.

There are names for men who like fat women, for women who like fat women, for fat women who like fat women. There is no name for women who like fat men. All the other variations are considered perverse. But fat men, like most men, are thought to be naturally attractive, to some women. Not to all. I had a Polish girlfriend in Paris who dropped me, she said, because I gained ten pounds. They made the difference in her eyes between being big and being fat.

* *Saint Louis Post-Dispatch,* January 7, 1995.

Marlon Brando is the most spectacular example of a man who has grown monstrously fat while remaining a sexual object. Brando is reported by his biographers to have had women abundantly at his disposal in years when his weight started rising above 240 pounds. In Tahiti, making *Mutiny on the Bounty,* he would sometimes get up and leave in the middle of shooting. He'd go out to the reef alone in a canoe, "maybe with a ten pound box of ice cream."[°] Keeping his refrigerator stocked was a full-time job for his housekeeper, Ray Ruysseveldt. When Brando arrived, he headed straight for the kitchen and "stuffed himself," sometimes with half a cheesecake, a pint of ice cream, or both. Karl Malden remembers how Brando would be on the set of *One-Eyed Jacks:* "Suddenly, we're eating and there it goes. Two steaks, potatoes, two apple pies à la mode, a quart of milk. I don't know what did it. Aggravation during the day maybe, but before you know it, they'd have to go out and make another outfit for him. He'd just bloat up."[†]

Brando would have his housekeepers padlock the refrigerator to keep him from consuming gallons of ice cream in the middle of the night. But while he was paying his help to keep him from eating, he would secretly pay other people to toss him food over the wall to feed his monstrous cravings.

Brando's success came despite the shame he felt about his fat. He was always putting off the nude scenes in *Last Tango in Paris.* "We have to wait a bit longer. I'm not thin enough yet," he would say.[‡] The diets never worked, so he ended up shooting the sex

---

[°] Peter Manso, *Brando: The Biography* (New York: Hyperion, 1994), p. 523.

[†] Ibid., p. 488.

[‡] Ibid., p. 242.

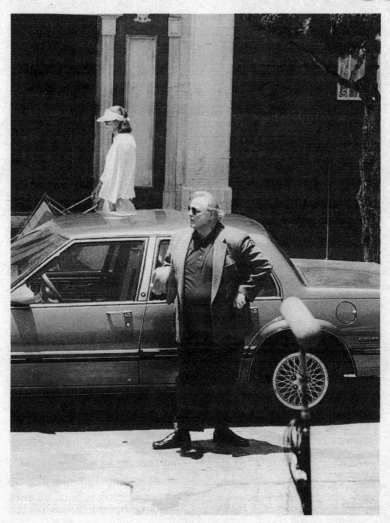

Marlon Brando

scenes either fully clothed or wearing an overcoat to conceal his naked girth. But Brando's shame goes hand in hand with a kind of boldness about transgressing the taboos we put on stuffing our bellies and blowing ourselves up.

M.F.K. Fisher, the great food writer, wrote:

> I cannot believe that there exists a single coherent human being who will not confess, at least to herself, that once or twice she had stuffed herself to the bursting point . . . for no other reason than the beastlike satisfaction of her belly. I pity anyone who has not permitted herself this sensual experience, if only to determine what her own private limitations are; and where, for herself alone, gourmandism ends and gluttony begins.*

The beastlike satisfaction of the belly is such a profoundly human, because deeply animal, impulse that Fisher feels pity for any human who has never let herself or himself be a bloated beast. Being an animal stuffed with food is the condition of being fully human, she says. You need once in a while to transgress the barrier between eating well and eating like a pig, in order to understand what eating well might mean. The church, of course, considers gluttony one of the cardinal sins. It would be a sin not to ever sin by gluttony, says M.F.K. Fisher. EAT

FAT means to eat well, to eat beautifully, even to eat slowly. It means, for example, to eat beef. Twenty

---

* M.F.K. Fisher, *An Alphabet for Gourmets* (New York: Viking Press, 1949), p. 16.

years ago eating beef was at a peak in this country; since then it's declined by about 25 percent. In the meantime, we've become a nation of bird eaters. Turkey and chicken have quadrupled in the same period. There certainly are indications that beef eating is back on the rise. Who knows why? A turn in the wheel of fashion or chicken fatigue? Humans can eat only so much chicken before they start getting sick of it.

Nevertheless we are still eating pretty much the same amount of fat. The average adult gets 34 percent of his or her calories from fat, and 12 percent of that from saturated fat. The consumption of fat has declined by just 2 percent since 1978, despite the fat-phobic propaganda. But who doesn't love the smell of steaks grilling in the air, the sizzle of a burger over flames as its sweet bloody pleasure takes prisoner of your nose and arouses all your buds to tingle and the saliva in us carnivores to flow.

EAT

FAT means, for example, eat chocolate. Sheila Lavery writes:

> Apparently, women need chocolate as well as other foods that are high in starch, sugar and fat to control weight, stabilize moods and revitalize well-being. Indeed, failing to satisfy these needs can lead to overeating, feelings of fatigue, frequent mood swings, debilitating premenstrual and menopausal symptoms, and uncontrollable food cravings.*

Women's bodies are genetically programmed to make fat; on the average, men have 12 percent less fat than women. Women

---

* "Why Women Need Chocolate," *Daily Mail*, February 16, 1995.

make fat more easily and release it more slowly than men do. It serves, among other things, the interest of the fetus to be surrounded by a nice fat cushion of nourishing fat—particularly if scarcity prowls. That may explain why women are often obsessed with chocolate; men rarely are. It appears women may need the fat in chocolate, sudden bursts of high energy to help lift moods and maintain metabolic functions. Most men don't really love chocolate, not the way a lot of women do—with a ferocious, compulsive love. Chocolate is a miraculous substance when it comes to providing the body with concentrated amounts of high fat and sugar.

We are a nation of chocoholics; in the United States, we spend more than $15 billion each year on the sweet stuff, while a recent Gallup survey showed that a third of women actually prefer chocolate to sex.* For most women to EAT

FAT would mean to eat chocolate. It might even be good for your health.

At Penn State, the researcher Yu-Yan Yeh and his student T. K. Pai reported that the saturated fat in beef and chocolate may not be so terrible after all. In fact it may help lower "bad" cholesterol. Rat liver cells were treated with fatty acids from palm oil and coconut oil, or with stearic acid from chocolate and meat. The latter resulted in much lower levels of triglyceride—a precursor to bad cholesterol.† It reminds you of Woody Allen's movie *Sleeper*, which takes place in an imagined future in which doctors, as always

* *London Daily Mail*, February 16, 1995.
† *Business Week*, May 1, 1995.

faddish, are recommending cigarettes and chocolate to their patients. They've discovered that they're good for your health.

But it is not in order to improve your health that this book suggests you EAT

FAT. It may happen, simply as a result of reading this book, that you find you have a healthier, happier, more casual relation to your food and your body—to the fat on the shelf and in the can. But there are no guarantees.

In particular, there are no individual guarantees. You have to entertain the real possibility that to change the beauty myth would require something like a political decision, a collective struggle, maybe even civil disobedience to resist the power of the idols of thin. This book wants to be a contribution to that struggle, helping to make it possible to think differently, or think anew, about what once was beautiful and may well be desirable again. Once the myth of beauty was fat. Now it's thin. It could certainly change again. It's not easy to change your image of what is beautiful and desirable, especially if those images have been programmed by your personal history, reinforced by the social environment, and manipulated by the cynical media.

It's all too easy these days to blame everything on television. But, on average, every child and adult in America watches television between four and five hours a day. A child who grows to maturity in our culture will have registered more millions of images than any child has ever seen in the history of the human race. Why does that fact alone not alarm us? Why at the moment are we so little suspicious of images? The Jewish religion is predicated on suspicion of graven images. There are none in synagogues. In the eastern church of Byzantium, there was a culture of illuminated icons, but the Western Roman Catholic church resisted the temptations of the image and, until the Renaissance, harbored a deep distrust of icons of all sorts, of painted images and representations, even in the theater, which it banned. Why? It was out of fear of idolatry. Today, we have no fear of idolatry—no anxiety about the power of images to confine our thoughts to the merely finite dimensions of what can be seen. The idolatry of images restricts our power to grasp possibilities that are hard to imagine but are nevertheless real. Creating idols, as in Hollywood, is one of America's principal export items. The world is being sold our images, and all those images are thin. The idols of the media these days are those superstars whose figures are anorexic.

Remember the emaciated woman on a swing in the ad, posing for a fashion benefit to support the National AIDS Fund? This, the ad tells us, is a *Vogue* Initiative.* What are we seeing here? Is this woman supposed to be a glamorous model, inviting us to a fashion show to benefit AIDS? Or is her desperate thinness a reminder of the emaciation attending the disease? I think she's supposed to be glamorous, but she illustrates, almost too well, what Naomi Wolf and others have taught us, that the ideal of glamour that we are being sold today is one in which women appear cadaverous. Like the woman on the trapeze, the idea of a fashionable woman is a creature suspended—helpless, weak, and vulnerable, arms and legs extended. Caught or frozen in the frame of the swing, like a butterfly skewered on the page, her little pigtails flapping on either side. She is so exposed in this picture

* Echoing protests in Britain, *Vogue* just announced its decision not to promote anorexic-looking models in its pages.

that instinctively she twists her left leg to displace the viewer's gaze from her exposed and ravished thinness. This is the beauty on behalf of which we are being invited to donate our money.

Who decided that women could not be fat and beautiful? Above all, without glamour. Glamour is distinguished from beauty in that it refers to the appearance of what is beautiful, to the presentation of what is perceived as an image of beauty. Something glamorous—presented by the media as beautiful—may strike many as not beautiful at all. Conversely, much beauty—perhaps the greatest—has no glamour. Even if fat were beautiful, it wouldn't be glamorous, not here, not now, not today. But it's been only ninety years since fat was adorable, and a hundred years before that, at the courts of Spain and France, thinness was an abomination.

Finding glamour in fat is not easy today, and maybe it's not a solution but part of the problem. Today, glamour has become an image tool, a brilliant aura with which markets can be manipulated, services rendered, products sold.

EAT

FAT means: Crush the images and crush the image-making machine. In order to see the beauty of fat it may be necessary to step outside the glamour machine, to refuse it, like old hippies or young punks do today, and look again. I haven't abandoned the dream of rearranging the grammar of glamour (the two words have the same root in Greek) in order to make fat glamorous. It won't be easy.

Comparatively speaking, I'm not very fat. My friends tell me or flatter me when I ask. I say, for example, Achh, I'm so fat. And they say, No, you're not fat. But I feel fat. I'm not. For a man of my age, I'm in decent enough shape. I run, do sit-ups, stretch, but when March rolls around, I've accumulated as much as 200 pounds on my 5' 8½" frame, before I stop looking at the scales. And then I'm really fat. My mother's side lent me a disposition to accumulate fat around my middle. That's the worst sort of fat, doctors say, since it impedes a lot of vital organs with a slick layer of grease that strains more than it lubricates. When I'm really fat, it all goes to my belly, which I can stick out and make seem immense. Most of the time I hold it in. The absence of any hips, combined with that familial tendency to accrete around the middle, makes me look pretty much like a pear when I'm up there.

I've been about 200 for some time, and I'm not happy. I need to lose 20 to 30 pounds.

At this moment, I'm statistically obese. Why lose? This is not a wish I occasionally muse about, this is a preoccupation that invades and engages my consciousness or my barely conscious states at least as many times a day as I put things into my mouth, which is often. In that respect I am like most Americans, according to one survey—preoccupied with their weight. Every time I am reminded I have a body, that I occupy actual space, that I am visible, I register the fat.

It seems clear to me, a man, that my constant dissatisfaction with my fat is nothing like what it would be if I were a woman. In fact, like a lot of men, there are times when I value and appreciate my fat. I don't feel it diminishes my appeal; it makes me feel bigger and stronger, more impressive and more serious. Down here in Florida, I see a lot of good old boys who flaunt their bellies and cultivate their paunch. But their appreciation of their own fat and other men's fat doesn't mean that they like it on women. Like them, but also differently, I've internalized forms of fat phobia.

I am reinforced by my mother and my sister, two fatties. They've both been dieting for decades, have been on quasi-permanent diets, and have been getting fatter and fatter. Like most people who diet. Like most of us—like me.

Suppose you were to decide to EAT

FAT and not be fat. It might be hard to do. But there are those who claim that the French do it all the time. Eskimos of course do it most of the time. It seems like an impossible ideal, contradictory, but it is the only one that *is* possible—that is worth trying to achieve. After years of blowing up and slimming down, I myself have only just begun to EAT

FAT. It's a process that this book wants to initiate. The results cannot be guaranteed. The process can only promise that if you follow this book, scrupulously, you will be exactly as fat as you want to be. My premise is not that we have but that we are our fat. It defines us; we shape it. Our fat sets the lines and the outlines of the space we occupy in the world with our bodies. It is a mirror of ourselves that no one ever sees directly—invisible beneath the skin, but visible in the contours of our form. The form of our fat makes us beautiful or ugly, in our own eyes or others'. It is, after our sex, the first thing the other registers concerning our identity, but unlike our gender it is idiosyncratic, specifically individual and unique, the molded shape of who we are.

Fat talks. It is the medium through which we communicate our body's messages to the world and by which we translate its imperatives and impositions onto our flesh. This book proposes to let you think about the way your fat talks—to you, about you, to others. It aims to free you to become the fat you are. EAT

FAT means, in the first place, to eat whatever you need, as much of it as you want, for as long as you like. How long do you think you'll gorge if you lift all restrictions on what you can eat. How soon would it be before you started putting limits on yourself? It gets expensive eating all the time. It takes time, shopping, shlepping, cooking. And after a while, your stomach revolts. At that point, either you have to kill the poor stomach, as Pavarotti did, or you cut back to what you normally would eat if you weren't always watching what you eat. Letting yourself eat what you want when you want it lets you start to discover the limits you want to put on your eating, rather than those that have been imposed on you by a guilty conscience. You start to invent a new economy of eating based on your own desires and needs to change the mood.

In the second place, it means you can start to discover your own proper fat. There is increasing evidence that each one of us has a given amount of fat that our body tries to maintain, against all the efforts to fatten or reduce it. It is that tendency of the body to over-react when weight is lost, to speed up its metabolism, or make fat more efficiently, that results in yo-yoing, blowing up after losing weight. EAT

FAT means to to restore the body's own conception of fine fat.

Finally, it means that fat is fair. This book, or at least its jacket, is there to remind you that it's been only in the last ninety years that thin has been considered beautiful. For most of human history, it's been fat that we found lovely to look at and delicious to feel, in our mouths or in our hands, pressed up against us, on the inside or the outside. It's possible that conditions are ripe for a change in attitudes that will result from a change in fashion. When full fat is fair again, when men and women love their fat, when fat is everywhere phat, then we fatties, who remember the old days, will laugh like lunatics free at last of the asylum.

Part One

THE WORD
FAT

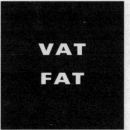

**VAT
FAT**

Fat, as we've already seen, originally meant vessel. So when you look up the word in the *Oxford English Dictionary*, the first definition is obsolete. The last documented use of the word in that sense occurs in 1866, but its roots go way back to Teutonic, the ancient language of what is now Germany—the mother of all the languages allied to and including modern German, the Scandinavian languages, and English. It was the language of Charlemagne and before that of the barbarous tribes that for the Romans became Germania—the country beyond the Rhine. °*Fat,* at its roots, is a verb meaning to hold, to contain, like a vessel or vat.

The high value that attaches to the word °*fat* arises not from the thing itself, but from what it contains. °*Fat* is precious because what it holds is very precious. In the church, the word °*fat* had a special meaning. It referred to slender silver vessels in which holy water was made portable and available to be sprinkled on altars and other places it sanctified. °*Fat* is precious and holy, because it contains what is blessed and procures blessings. The priest sprinkles holy water from a silver vessel that, like the church itself, is a reservoir of holiness that allows its blessing to be transported and distributed. Sometimes the °*fat* is yellow like gold: "The golden Fat out of which they take the water" is a phrase that appears in 1678, according to the *Oxford English Dictionary*. Next time you look in the mirror, think of your fat as a golden °*fat* containing holy water.

The more general sense of °*fat* was of a large-size vessel for liquids, a tub, a dyer's or a brewer's vat, a wine cask, and especially the tub or vat in which wine was pressed by stamping feet. A °*fat,* a fat vat, is the happiest vat in life. In it men and women, grape harvesters, culminate and celebrate their whole year of hard work, in a well-oiled dance over the newly picked grapes, on which hopes for so much future intoxication, joy, and warmth depend. In 1593, Arthur Golding, in his translation of Ovid's *Metamorphoses,* wrote of "Harvest smeared with treading grapes late at the pressing fat." The pressing fat is the vat in which you smear yourself with grapes; in celebration of cornucopian abundance, you cover yourself with the harvested fruit, impregnating yourself, inside and out, with the purple prose of intoxication. The grape vat is a dyer's vat in which the celebrants bathe, totally immersing themselves in this bacchic baptism. Look in the mirror and think of your fat as a great cask, a °*fat* for stomping on grapes. Repeat the word °*fat* to yourself slowly, and think of the charm the word must have had for our ancestors the Teutons, gathered for the harvest at the °*fat.*

Shakespeare uses fat to mean vat in *Antony and Cleopatra,* when the Roman general worries about losing his martial enthusiasm in the luxury of Cleopatra's court. He says to her, "In thy fats our cares be drowned" (II, vii, 122). He doesn't mean he'll drown in her fat, but in her wine barrels. Although Cleopatra herself is a vessel containing infinite amounts of pleasure, unimagined beauty, and ancient secrets, like wine, she makes generals lose their heads. In her body, in her fat, Antony will drink and lose himself. The °*fats* of Cleopatra are the emblem of what one critic calls "the opposition of fat and effeminating Egypt to lean and virile Rome in Shakespeare's *Antony and Cleopatra.*"° A little earlier Pompey proposes to draw lots to see which of them will be the first to give a banquet celebrating their alliance. Antony declines to choose, but Pompey insists, teasing him for having tasted too deeply at the banquet tables of Egypt.

> *Pompey.* No, Antony, take the lot: but first
> Or last, your fine Egyptian cookery
> Shall have the fame. I have heard that Julius Caesar
> Grew fat with feasting there. [II, vi, 63]

By referring to Caesar's growing fat, Pompey is slyly evoking Cleopatra, who was Caesar's mistress before she became Antony's. The opposition between virile Rome and effeminate Egypt is epitomized by the couch of Cleopatra, on which all these Romans dream of making love, eating, drinking, and getting fat. Caesar's fat,

---

° Patricia Parker, *Literary Fat Ladies: rhetoric, gender, property* (London: Methuen, 1987), p. 14.

like Mark Antony's, is more than just an extra roll of flab; it represents the accumulation of a universe of pleasure so vast and deep that it can totally transform the character of even the leanest Roman centurion. If Caesar can, why not grow fat with feasting?

There's an old proverb repeated in Bunyan's *Pilgrim's Progress* that goes, "Every fat must stand on its own bottom." Allegorically it means that each person should act on his own behalf, independently. A vat's bottom, a °*fat* bottom, must stand alone, to keep what it contains from seeping or leaking, to prevent any confusion of vats. Even today, the same meaning is used in a figurative sense when different schools within a single university are treated for budgetary purposes as distinct and separate "tubs." The law school, the engineering school, arts and sciences, each stands on its own, on its own bottom. Fat bottoms are what guarantee the purity and the unity of whatever is supposed to go together in a single tub. Fat stands on its own bottom, independent, self-contained, held together by its own sense of integrity, of separate independence from others. Next time you look at your fat bottom, think of what a sense of grounding it provides.

What's cute about tubby? TUBBY! The letter *B*, of course, is fat, so you have two big bursting bellies sticking out in tubby. But it's true as well that when a ship is derisively called a tub, it's too broad for its length. A tubby person is similarly wider than higher, and like most tubs a likely butt of humor.

Like a ton, a fat of something is a measure that equals 9 gallons. Ton, by the way, comes from *tonne*, which in French means a big barrel, or tub. Fat always refers to an amount, to the condition of there being an accumulated amount of something. As a noun, fat

first meant vat, but as an adjective it has always referred in general
to the bulk or condition of things.

In its earliest use as an adjective, in its current sense, *fat* means
ready to be killed, well fed, well supplied with fat. In the fourteenth
century, Wycliff's translation of the Bible spoke of "a feste of fatte
bestes"—that is, a feast of fat beasts. Something fat means it's good
enough to eat. Something lean is fattened up until it's well supplied
with fat and ripe for the butcher. But ripe can also mean sexy and
ready to trot, as when Falstaff, all hot and bothered, is waiting for
love in Windsor wood: "For me," he says, "I am here a Windsor
stag; and the fattest, I think, i' the forest." It's the middle of the
summer, hot as hell, and Falstaff is fat and hot enough already. He
calls on Jupiter to cool it down, this mating season, otherwise he's
going to start to melt and piss wax. "Send me a cool rut-time, Jove,
or who can blame me to piss my tallow? Who comes here? my
doe?" (*The Merry Wives of Windsor,* V, v, 14.) Fat is wax, and fat
tends to wax, or grow. As Francis Bacon, in *Sylva Sylvorum, a natural historie,* observes, "The Bear, the Hedgehog . . . wax fat when
they Sleep." Fat grows fatter just by doing nothing. All by itself fat
has a natural tendency to increase, no disposition to decline.

Even the meaning of fat waxes. According to the *Oxford
English Dictionary,* the word, used as an adjective, originally meant
well supplied with fat, but almost immediately, very early, it begins
to mean very well supplied, oversupplied, corpulent, obese, with
connotations that are clearly pejorative. It's an old story. When Falstaff dresses as a woman he becomes "an old woman, a fat woman,"
"an old fat woman" (*Wives,* IV, v). Shakespeare writes of "a fat
rogue," "a gross fat man," "ye fat paunch" (*Henry IV: Part I,* I, ii,

18); "fat rascals," "fat villain," "that fat belly of his" (*Henry IV: Part II,* II, iiii, 4); "fat paunches have lean pates" (*Love's Labour's Lost,* I, i, 2): fat men are bald. But a fat bald man like Falstaff can use fat as a flattering adjective to describe the loveliest thing in the world that a rogue and a thief can imagine: "There are traders riding to London with fat purses" (*Henry IV: Part I,* I, ii, 141).

"Fat purses" is an expression in which fat is used both literally and metaphorically. The purse itself is pumped up, plump and full of gold coins, but a fat purse, like a fat kitchen, is a rich one, well stocked. The literal fatness on the outside, the rounded plumpness of the purse, stands for the metaphorical fatness, the abundant riches, on the inside. It's in a literal sense that olives are fat and oily, that fat cheese is unctious and tender; fat milk makes cream, fat broth is thick, and a fat goose is maybe the fattest thing of all to eat. A serving of goose stuffed with foie gras, in the classic preparation, is reported to be about 4,225 calories per person, according to a French cookbook, designed for people who love fat and want to gain weight, called *Be Both Fat and Beautiful.*°

Take a well-fatted twelve-pound goose. Chop its liver and heart together with another fresh goose liver. Mix this together with slices of truffle, some parsley, and a dash of Armagnac. Stuff the goose with this mixture, whose richness of flavor and intensity of odor belong to some tragic essence of dark, rich, fat food. I make a version of this recipe myself in upstate New York with many fewer resources than those of M. Laffiteau. Instead of the fresh foie gras

° Cyril Laffiteau, *Gros et beau à la fois* (*Be Both Fat and Beautiful*) (Levallois-Perret: Editions Filipacchi, 1995), p. 57.

the recipe calls for, I buy the best canned pâté I can find. In the absence of fresh truffle, I shell out for a tiny can of a meager one shrunk to the size of a black marble. I shave the truffle, mix it together with the pâté, a little parsley, and, short of Armagnac, a shot of the best brandy I can get. Finally, you take some plump, pitted prunes and fill them carefully with this mixture. When that's done (it takes some time), I stuff the fat goose with the filled prunes that are stuffed with liver studded with truffles, perfumed by the liquor of the heavy southern grapes of Périgord. To summon up in imagination the poetic power—the profundity of flavored fatness—this dish exudes, consider the corresponding analogies: liver is to meat, as goose is to fowl, as prune is to fruit. Each one, in its own separate domain, belongs to the pole of what is dark, and deep, and richly delicious, fatted and fattening, beyond belief. This dark fat is sublime shit. In America, Fat shit! is no big deal, but the French, when speaking about some fat Burgundy or a golden Armagnac often say that is has the faint but unmistakable scent of pig *merde*—and that is very good.

A fat room is one full of dense air, thick and fat with moistures of love. "Come out of that fat room," says Prince Hal to Poins, when he tears him away from the lubricious pleasures of women's flesh and fat beer suffusing the tavern (*Henry IV: Part I*, II, iv, 1).

Fat land has fat soil; fat fields are fruitful and fertile. A fat living or a fat job is a good one: lawyers like to try a fat case; printers, paid by the page, prefer a fat one—a page of print that's mostly blank, widely spaced, with few lines and little type. A fat kingdom has fat pastures where people eating off the fat of the land are fat with feasting. Caesar says, "Let me have men about me that are fat"

(*Julius Caesar,* I, ii, 19). Conversely, men who have a "lean and hungry look," like Cassius, harbor hollow souls and sinister ambitions.

Shakespeare uses the word *fat* at least seventy times in his work. It is one of the signs of the abjection into which fat has fallen, that the flattering meanings of the word have been lost in the present rush to despise it. Shakespeare takes fat to metaphorical extremes of excellence. He writes of the "fat ribs of peace" (*King John,* III, iii) and the "fat rump and potato finger" of luxury, "the fat earth's store" (*The Rape of Lucrece,* 183). He stretches the adverb and verb *fat* to the furthest extremes of their figural meaning. "I will feed fat the ancient grudge I bear him" (*The Merchant of Venice,* V, i, 3). And "Advantage feeds him fat, while men delay" (*Henry IV: Part I,* III, ii, 18). In the expression "feed fat," the word is used as an adverb to mean abundantly, richly, just as "eat fat" can be heard to mean to eat well. Feeding fat and eating fat are intimately joined. Did you know there's a hot line, a 900 number, you can call to meet Encouragers and Gainers, those who feed fat and those who eat fat, people whose whole sexual life centers on gaining weight and helping others put it on? Does the sexual pleasure you get from feeding other people fat equal in intensity that received from eating fat and growing it?

The verb *fat* appears several times in Shakespeare, as in "Would they but fat their thoughts with this? (*Troilus and Cressida,* II, ii, 4.) But the most famous instance is in *Hamlet.* When the king asks, "Where's Polonius?" the prince, having just stabbed and killed the old politician concealed behind a curtain, answers, "At supper."

"At supper!" [exclaims the king.] "Where?"
Hamlet. Not where he eats, but where he is eaten. A certain

convocation of politic worms are e'en at him. Your worm is your
only emperor for diet. We fat all creatures else to fat us, and we
fat ourselves for maggots. Your fat king and your lean beggar is
but variable service, two dishes, but to one table.
That's the end. [IV, iii, 18–26]

Polonius, beneath the ground, is at supper, but it's he who is being
eaten by political worms, those that eat politicians for lunch and
supper. Worms, says Hamlet, are the last emperors of diet, the mas-
ters of the great fat chain of being, those creatures for whom all
food is finally, ultimately intended. We fatten all creatures to fat
ourselves; we fat ourselves to fatten maggots, the last fed fat. Fat
kings and thin beggars alike feed worms, and therefore, despite all
the difference in the dignity and quantity of their fat, they humbly
serve the same end, the same last supper.

A whole book has been written titled *Literary Fat Ladies*, by
Patricia Parker who begins her survey in the Bible with the figure
of Rahab, the fat whore of Jericho, who redeemed herself, betraying the heathens and embracing the Israelites, by letting them into
the Promised Land. Her conversion meant, says Parker, that she
went from "letting in men to letting in men": from whore to gate-
keeper, opening her gates. Her name, which in Hebrew means
"broad" or "wide," was translated by the Church Fathers as *dilatio:*
opening, expanding. She got taken up in the Middle Ages and interpreted, not surprisingly, as a figure of the church itself. The church,
another redeemed harlot, expands to fill the time between the First
and Second Coming, letting in those she loves and keeping others
out. During the long interval, the much deferred postponement of
the apocalyptic end of time, this whore dilates, opening to receive

more and more humanity, but also in this time to dilate or propa-
gate the Word. "The dilation of Rahab or of the Church, then,
involves symbolically two orifices," says Parker.° Rahab is not only a
whore, she's a female, and so according to the oldest rag of misog-
yny, she can't keep either orifice shut. This fat lady won't shut up;
she's fat and voluble, with a swelling, fleshy style, full of verbal
interlarding, obeying the principle of increase. And once she loses
her religious associations, in the Renaissance, she becomes a
rotund figure of romance. In literature, fat and bawdy ladies, like
the Wife of Bath in Chaucer, tell tall tales: "My jolly body shall a tale
tell," the Wife says, whose motto is "increase and multiply."†

One of the great fat ladies in Shakespeare is Nell in *The Com-
edy of Errors,* whom we never actually see. She is described by
Dromio of Syracuse, who has been fending off her advances. She's
"a wondrous fat marriage," he tells Antipholus, by which he means
"she's the kitchen wench, and all grease." But grease is next to
grace, so she's "a very reverent body." Like a stubby candle, she's
made of so much greasy tallow she'd "burn a Poland winter." "If
she lives till doomsday, she'll burn a week longer than the whole
world" (III, ii). She's lubricious, lewd, and well-lubed; she's glossy,
chubby, and hot.

Grace is grease. A graceful dancer slips across the floor, flows
easily with the liquid smoothness, the frictionless effort of what is
suave, fluent, polished, and fine. The fat, it's often been noted, are
good dancers, smooth and graceful as silky grease.

° Parker, p. 14.
† Ibid., p. 16.

Nell, this kitchen wench, is round, "No longer from head to foot than from hip to hip. She is spherical, like a globe." And being a globe, her body offers continents of flesh to the avid explorer, and smaller zones as well. "I could find out countries in her," says Dromio of Syracuse (III, ii).

> *Antipholus.* In what part of her body stands Ireland?
> *Dromio S.* Marry, sir, in her buttocks; I found it out by the bogs.

(A bog, of course, is wet spongy ground, a mossy morass, over which travelers pass and sometimes sink.)

> *Antipholus.* Where stood Belgia, the Netherlands?
> *Dromio S.* Oh, sir, I did not look so low. [III, ii]

But the fattest lady in Shakespeare is not a lady but a knight, Sir John Falstaff, who in *The Merry Wives of Windsor* appears dressed as a woman. The play was written at the behest of Queen Elizabeth herself, who couldn't get enough of the bard's great comic creation who twice already, in *Henry IV*, Parts I and II, had gaudily stolen the show. His name suggests that, being so fat and voluble, he has always been somewhat effeminized, missing something manly, a Fall-staff, as Parker observes.* These days, as has been observed, fat makes men effeminate but gives women virile substance. Like other literary fat ladies, Falstaff is "a hill of flesh," "a globe of sinful continents." He's an inexhaustible cornucopia of verbosity and of

---

* Ibid., p. 20.

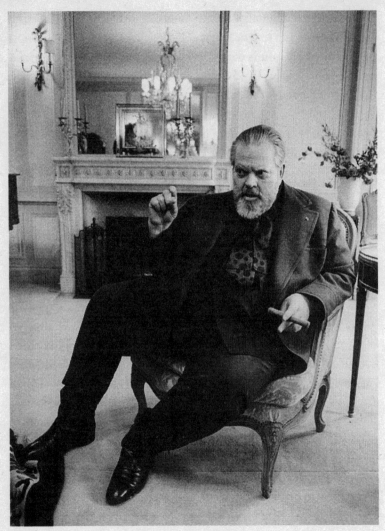

Orson Welles

flesh, a figure of dilation who "lards the lean earth as he walks along" but never gets to the point; in short, "a sweet creature of bumbast."° The pun is that bombast refers literally to cotton wool used as padding or stuffing for clothes, as well as figuratively to orotund, inflated language.

Falstaff says, "I was born about three in the afternoon, with a white head and something of a round belly." W. H. Auden tries to connect the infant belly of Falstaff with the "drinker's belly he so prominently develops in old age." Auden writes,

> If one visits a bathing beach, one can observe that men and women grow fat in different ways. A fat woman exaggerates her femininity; her breasts and buttocks enlarge till she comes to look like the Venus of Willendorf. A fat man, on the other hand, looks like a cross between a very young child and a pregnant mother. There have been cultures in which obesity in women was considered the ideal of sexual attraction, but in no culture, so far as I know, has a fat man been considered more attractive than a thin one. I would say that fatness in the male is the physical expression of a psychological wish to withdraw from sexual competition and, by combining mother and child in his own person, to become emotionally self-sufficient. The Greeks thought of Narcissus as a slender youth but I think they were wrong. I see him as a middle-aged man with a corporation, for, however ashamed he may be of displaying it in public, in private a man with a belly loves it dearly; it may be

° Ibid.

an unprepossessing child to look at, but he has borne it all by himself.[*]

Auden reminds us that a "corporation," vulgarly speaking, is a big gut. We call it a beer belly, but, according to the *Oxford English Dictionary*, in 1813 Smollett proudly, patriotically propounds of his paunch, "Sirrah! my corporation is made up of good wholesome English fat." Grose's *A Classical Dictinary of the Vulgar Tongue* (1785) gives "He has a glorious corporation," and Charlotte Brontë in *Shirley* writes of the "dignity of an ample corporation."[†] This meaning seems quaint today, but it might be useful to revive it as a way of thinking about what we call corporations in the 1990s; like their anatomical counterparts, these great abdomens seem to aim only at expanding, greedily incorporating and consolidating in view of increasing their volume, enlarging their scale, heightening visibility, and enhancing prestige.

It seems odd that Auden says that no culture has ever found fat men more attractive than thin ones. That seems very odd when you think of Tonga, or West Germany after the war, or America in the Gay Nineties, or certain gay bear bars in London, or when you think of Santa Claus. No culture has ever preferred a thin to a fat Santa Claus. Maybe Auden's error is a gay thing; mainstream gay homosexual culture is, or used to be, even more fat phobic than so-called heterosexual culture, however hard that is to believe.

---

[*] W. H. Auden, *The Dyer's Hand and Other Essays* (New York: Vintage, 1968), pp. 195–96.

[†] *Oxford English Dictionary*, under the word *corporation*, sense #6.

Auden doesn't like fat. He castigates those people, mostly drinkers with fat bellies (like himself), who flee from adult responsibilities and opt out of sexual competition. They are seeking, he says, "some means to become again the Falstaffs they once were." We were all Falstaffs when we were children, greedily sucking on life, totally self-absorbed, with no moral purpose, only the inexhaustible desire that our own importance be acknowledged by others with the same fervor that we recognize it ourselves. A man who drinks and gets fat is, therefore, in Auden's view, an escapist back to that condition of infantile self-absorption. Growing fat, he says, we embody simultaneously the mother and the child, the child wrapped in the fat cocoon of the mother's hovering attention, whose love is indistinguishable from the narcissistic attention the child pays himself. Mother and child are self-contained in the perfect sphere of a big gut.

Auden, in a note, tries to bring some clarity to these formulations. He nuances his bald claims: "Not all fat men are heavy drinkers, but all males who drink heavily become fat [note: All the women I have met who drank heavily were lighter and thinner than average]."[*]

In *Hamlet* there is an often overlooked line, which appears in the mouth of Gertrude, the queen, in the last scene of the play. Hamlet is returning from dueling and as he enters, his mother observes, "He is fat and scant of breath." Laura Keyes has shown how difficult it is for modern audiences to accept the idea that Hamlet is fat, even if his name points to that fat fact.[*] Ham-let is a

[*] Auden, p. 196.

ham, a porky piggy hogger of the limelight, a bad actor who can't tell the stage from reality. Once you realize that fact and start looking for fat, you quickly discover it everywhere in the play. Who can stop laughing when, in Act I, scene ii, Hamlet steps forth alone to the front of the stage and prays:

> Oh, that this too too solid flesh would melt,
> Thaw, and resolve itself into a dew!

It's as if he's giving eternal expression to the deathless dream of everyone who ever wanted to lose a few pounds.

A fat Hamlet is funny. Why? Because we prefer to attribute Hamlet's heroic indecision to noble motives, not to the low encumbrances of fat flesh. It's funny to think that what makes Hamlet tough to move when the going gets tough may be nothing more than the "non-executive or lymphatic temperament" with which we stigmatize the fat—the moral consequences of their lack of breath and fatty deposits around the heart [Keyes 90]. All the talk about avenging his father's murder succumbs to the inertia of his avoirdupois. A fat Hamlet poses a contradiction between the mecurial fleetness of his witty reflections and the bulk of his breathless blubber.

But Keyes quotes one critic who defends the dramatic truth of Hamlet's fat. Hamlet, he writes, "is a robust soldier, accustomed to manly exercise, but a trifle out of form owing to his sojourn at the

---

° "Hamlet's Fat," in Sidney Homan, ed., *Shakespeare and the Triple Play: From Study to Stage to Classroom* (Lewisburg, Pa.: Bucknell University Press, 1988).

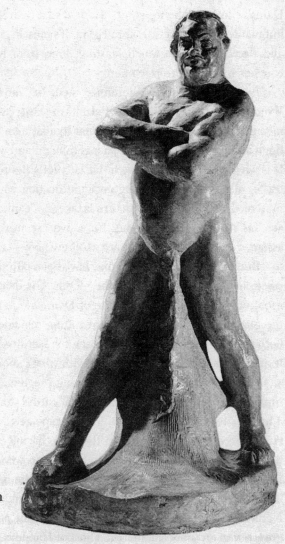

Balzac by Rodin

Danish court, and hence stout." Hamlet's fat then is not ridiculous, but manly, like that of Caesar in Egypt; it's muscle grown a little soft and flaccid from too much feasting, limp from lying around on couches with dangerous women.

But fat also used to effeminize men. In *The Merry Wives of Windsor*, Shakespeare puts fat Falstaff in skirts, as if, for men, fat meant always being in drag. Men fear it; a fat man is flabby, soft at thigh and breast and belly. Or so it is thought and written by some. It is what allows critics to see in fat Hamlet a figure of male impotence, of castration, implying an identification with Gertrude his mother. That identification in turn is taken to "explain" his failure to act, his reluctance to assume the active executive role normally assigned to men. Fat Hamlet is a Mommy's boy—a sort of girl.

But if Hamlet were fat, he may have been fatted for a ritual sacrifice, in which he himself is the victim. His death is a sacrifice required to purify the rotten state of Denmark, in order to permit the birth of one newly cleansed of rotting regicide. His fatness is both the sign that he has been chosen for sacrifice and an index of fertility: about to die, he's pregnant with what's about to be born.

Growing fat frequently means being pregnant, fertile, or nurturing, as in "Fair sun that breeds the fat earth's store." The earth is a mother fertilized by the sun, in Shakespeare's *Rape of Lucrece* [183]. Or when Hamlet says to the king, having just killed Polonious: "We fat all creatures else to fat us, and we fat ourselves for maggots" [4.03]. And that constant cycle of fattening and eating fat is the food cycle itself, the circle of life—of humans inserted into Nature. To fatten in Elizabethan speech meant not only to make grow but to grow succulent. The ghost of Hamlet's father speaks to his son from beyond the grave about the "fat weed" that grows on the shores of Lethe, the river of forgetfulness. It sounds like a good cigar, or a fat joint, one that is rolled thick, tastes delicious and dulls memory.

FAT FREE

Let me express the rage I feel toward the word *obesity*. This ugly noun, with all its pejorative implications, this term for unhealthy corpulence, has been mobilized by the medical-health-beauty industry, and wielded by food packagers, in order to stigmatize people who don't conform to an absurdly restrictive concept of ideal weight. Whereas fat is a good Anglo-Saxon word, obese comes from the Latin *obesus*, "having eaten well," past participle of *obedere*, to eat thoroughly, to devour, to chow down. The noun *obesity*, rare before the nineteenth century, had a sinister rebirth in popularity under the pen, in the hands of nineteenth-century doctors and health workers, medical imperialists seeking to police bodies by policing the language with which one might once have referred, for example, to someone's embonpointment.

The alternative to obesity, the image of the thin body beautiful and the ideal of health it promotes, is an ideological construct, a false nature, conceived by a vast industry in order to sell its services and move its products. Removing fat, the latest medical fad (does anyone think it won't soon be something else?), eliminates one more pleasure from our diet. After alcohol and tobacco, now fat has been proscribed. America, under the spur of its persistent Puritanism, cruelly medicalizes the matter of public health and social morality, of disease and compulsion. The health industry has already deemed food to be medicine, and fat is poison. That industry, with its ally, the government, is about to turn fat into a drug, which will give it the absolute control it desires, not only over occasional pleasures, like tobacco or liquor, but over food itself, which has the peculiarly profitable quality, distinct from that of any other drug, of being indispensable to life. The drumbeat of moralizing around food is rising to feverish intensity. But why then is everybody so fat? And getting fatter?

My hypothesis is this: If marketers can create guilt in a population saturated in fat, they can use obesity to sell both health and unhealth. Two messages, simultaneous, contradictory, very effective: The ostensible message is eat no fat; the cynical, maybe unconscious, one is EAT.

Go to a supermarket and try to find some fat. From the shelves everything screams, "NO FAT." The din it makes implies that the shoppers, the consumers of this message, must be mostly fat. They are. The rule seems to be this: The more no fat, the more fat. No fat authorizes eating more.

No Fat. Without Fat. Low Fat, Lo, Less Fat, 0g fat, no unsaturated fat, no cholesterol. Fat Free or, more and more often, just

FREE. Sometimes you even see New Free, the two words advertisers love most.

The more fat free the better, which means the more it lacks the more it's worth. The supermarket shelves display a whole hierarchy of lack that goes from no fat, to low or lo fat, to less fat, or fewer calories, or the complex litote of "I Can't Believe It's Not Butter!" which advertises that it has "50% less Fat and calories than butter and margarine." It's not exactly good for you, but eat and enjoy; it could be twice as bad. It actually comes in two forms, the regular and the "I Can't Believe It's Not Butter! Light." The question is: Who is speaking here? The consumer who hasn't tried it yet? She's buying a product whose name tells her what she's going to exclaim when she puts it in her mouth. Or maybe it's the product itself speaking to us as we pass its shelf. Not even it can believe that it isn't butter; it implies in taste, we hear in fat.

THE POEM OF NO FAT

Fleischmann's Lower Fat Margarine
No saturated fat
0mg cholesterol
Ingredient: Partially hydrogenated corn oil

Parkay Spread
Less fat and calories than margarine
70% less saturated fat than butter

LAND O LAKES Margarine
30% less saturated fat than leading margarines

Light Butter

Jell-O Fat Free Pudding Snacks

Uncle B's Bagels
Low fat, no cholesterol

Low Fat Muffins

Fat free
Healthy Choice
Non fat cream cheese

Breakstone's Fat Free Sour Cream
Now fat free

Kraft Favorites Fat Free
Shredded non-fat cheddar cheese
50 calories per serving
Low cholesterol
Ingredients: pasteurized skim milk and milk**
    **trivial source of fat

Healthy Choice Low Fat
Beef Franks
90% Fat free

Shofar Lite Kosher
Beef Frankfurters

Swift Premium
Pork and Turkey
Sizzlean

Breakfast, Lunch, and Dinner Strips
50% Less Fat
than bacon before heating

Jones Braunschweiger Liverwurst Lite
60% less fat
50% fewer calories
than the average Braunschweiger, USDA HB 8-7
Ingredients: Pork liver, pork and bacon

Miracle Whip
FREE
Non-fat dressing

Betty Crocker's
Bac-O's Chips
no cholesterol
partially hydrogenated soy oil

Hormel's Real Bacon Bits
50% less fat

Nabisco's Fat-Free Fig Newtons

Health Valley's Fat Free Healthy
Chocolate Cookies with Strawberry Centers
"These cookies promote good health . . ."
1 serving (about 2 cookies) 80 calories

Ultra Slim Fast
Peanut Butter Crunch
40% less fat than the leading candy bars
"Lose weight, feel great"

Weight Watchers
Smart Snackers Cheese Curls
45% less fat than comparable snacks

Healthy Choice Low Fat Smoked Sausage

Mrs. T's
Low Fat Frozen Pierogies

MORNINGSTAR Farm's Scramblers
Cholesterol Free
Egg Product
With Artificial Egg Flavor

Hostess Lights
Low Fat Twinkies

Sealtest Free
Fat free
Eskimo Pie
sweetened with Nutrisweet

Healthy Choice Malt Caramel Cone
Premium Low Fat Ice Cream

Dannon Pure Indulgence
Frozen yogurt

Pudding Bars
97% fat free

Hormel SPAM Lite

Look at what it says on a bag of Frito-Lays New Baked Tostitos: "Our oven baked chips let you indulge in more snacking fun . . . great taste without guilt. In fact, they have only one gram of fat per serving." A double message: Eat me, you eat less, so eat more and more of me, by way of snacking fun, for the sake of pure recreation, of repetitive putting hand to mouth—a handful of the nuts and chips and chocolates and snacks that fill our lives. More snacking fun . . . great taste without guilt. Ordinarily, sure, great taste and great guilt go together, particularly in this culture. Ordinarily if you go buy a bag of Tostitos, you think, No! That's fat. I'm here in this market sort of in order to cheat on my diet, but I cannot let myself do Tostitos. But these Tostitos are, more or less, less fat than ordinary chips. Eat, eat—I've just made a wonderful decision to eat what I might have passed up—snacking fun I would have missed. Do marketing strategies like these promote health in our society? Or obesity? The answer of course is both, and it works very well, thank you. Except that we keep on getting fatter.

What is interesting to observe in the supermarket is the ingenuity with which language is used to sell what in principle ought not be sellable. Consider the plight of commodities not blessed with no fat; bacon, for example, has a problem selling itself in the present environment. If not fat free, but if fat in fact, like bacon, it can only represent itself as being less than something more purely what it is. Swift Premium Pork and Turkey, Lunch, and Dinner Strips, to illustrate, has "50% Less Fat than bacon before heating." The virtue of this is obscure, since you're never ever going to eat your bacon raw.

The advertisers exploit the ambiguity of the word *less*, which normally indicates that some comparison is being made but which in English can stand alone, bearing only an implied comparison with something else taken to be the essence or norm of the thing. You don't have to know less fat than what, to be stirred by the appeal of "Less Fat."

Less fat means more eating, because the eating is without guilt, hence more pleasurable, hence more willingly entered into. Nabisco's Snack Well's Double Fudge Cookie Cake is "Fat Free." And, on its label, it says that it "tastes so great you'll never miss the fat." You are being reminded of what they would like you to forget, that you'll miss the fat. You will. And you will probably eat more of something else to compensate. The strategy is one that Roland Barthes often analyzed in *Mythologies;* the advertiser anticipates the consumer's negative reactions in order to make them explicit and soften their force of resistance.

By turning food into a drug, food can serve both as a poison to be controlled and a medicine to be dispensed. Health Valley may make excellent products, but consider the way it uses statistics, provided by the health industry, to inform and entice its consumers. It tells nothing but the truth, as the truth has been most officially, reliably determined:

Why this Fat-Free Chili is better for you.
This chili helps you fulfill the published dietary guidelines of the American Heart Association and the National Cancer Society. It is fat-free, with no cholesterol. One serving provides 10% of the U.S. RDA of protein, 15% of iron, and 100% of vitamin A in the form of beta-carotene. Beta-carotene is recommended by health experts as a key nutrient for main-

taining good health. And it contains over 50% less salt than leading chilis. So you can use this chili as part of a healthy diet that may help reduce your risk of heart disease and certain forms of cancer.

I rage at this when I see my mother eating this chili filled out with chopped meat, enhanced by cheese, probably salt. It's all right, though, she says to herself. She isn't exactly eating the chili; she's being helped to fulfill dietary guidelines. The more she eats, the more she gets of the good medicine it dispenses in the precisely measured, officially approved quantities of the U.S. RDA, the United States Recommended Daily Allowances, especially of beta-carotene, recommended by "health experts" (until last month). The more she eats of this good stuff, the more she helps reduce her risk of heart disease and cancer. She has been lured by the truth on the label into believing she's on the road to getting thinner, while she's getting fatter. Her example confirms what a researcher in Philadelphia claims to have discovered, scientifically—that if people are told food is lower in fat, they tend to eat more of it than they normally would.°

Entrancing shelves of supermarkets are awash with facts on labels, blanketed in blizzards of numbers, statistical percentages prominently displayed. FDA labeling requirements are located strategically on packaging to misdirect attention, deflect interest, induce boredom, mitigate evidence, in order to insinuate values, enhance claims, or boldly proclaim true facts or figures that can be connected together to paint a misleading picture of health.

° *U.S. News and World Report,* May 16, 1994.

The psychology that motivates the allure of food as medicine is succinctly stated on the package of some Italian biscuits:

NO-NO
"is a yes-yes"
New All Natural Biscotti
Fat Free Coconut

No-no is a yes-yes pretty much sums up the rhetorical strategy that generates the extraordinary profusion of figures and forms that sells food in our markets. Like a sexual harasser, the consumer doesn't have to take no for an answer. He can persuade himself that no is yes: a desire that ought to be resisted can be guiltlessly indulged. "Eating fat can make you fat," it says on the chili can. But it neglects to add that eating nothing but fat doesn't necessarily make you obese; look at Eskimos. It's not eating fat that makes you fat, it's eating. The chili says, eat me: No fat in my can, no fat on yours. Of course, there may be circumstances when eating no fat means being thin, but the chili-can label creates the illusion that there is some immediate equivalence between this fat and that, between no fat here and no fat there. In fact, eating too much fat-free chili will make you fat.

I say, NO MORE OBESITY. Let's hear it a while for fat.

Hold up, for example, Orson Welles. He was obese. But I praise his fat, I love his fat, I am grateful for the taste and energy and generosity, toward himself and others, that went into his accumulating that fat. Or I think of Roland Barthes, the great French critic, whose vast stomach I used to watch in class and admire; it took him a lifetime, cruelly abbreviated (not by cardiac arrest but by a truck), to acquire that paunch, an eternity of sitting—sitting reading, above all. But also writing and painting and eating and mostly everything else. Barthes never dreamed of exercise.

Take Pavarotti. I honor his fat, I admire the sacrifice and will required to make his body into the ennobling instrument it is. Every pound of his fat has my utter respect. I mean that. Or take Roseanne. That is one fat lady I would not kick out of my bed. I salute her for being a kind of heroine of her class, reminding suburbia that working-class people have reasons, perhaps, to be more "obese" than rich people, and that fat is sexy.

Face it. Who doesn't dream about great pools of yellow, oleaginous streams of liquid fat spreading its gentle balm over rough surfaces, smoothing hurts and filling up the painful spaces in things? Fat lends flavor to life, the flavor of everything that smoothly melts in your mouth, that creams into liquid pleasure. Food is the foremost pleasure left to those who despair of having sex. In the age of AIDS, as sex becomes more fraught with dangers, real and imaginary, food increasingly permits the displacement of libidinal cathexis—the flow of sexual energy—into substitute gratification. And food, in this country, is every day becoming more explicitly sexy. Ask the foodies. Gael Greene writes restaurant reviews that make you think of her heroines eating food off the bodies of their lovers; Sheila Lukens is photographed lying on a table, satyrically lowering a bunch of grapes to her deliciously parted lips. There is every reason to expect that the spreading of lo/no fat, with its tasteless blandness, will create in time great national cravings for the pleasure of food, orgies and banquets on a vast scale.

A lot of women love fat men. It's surprising how many are willing to avow the strength of their attraction to men like the late Raymond Burr, when he's Perry Mason, or to John Goodman, when he's Dan. They often fantasize the pleasure of being crushed by a big man, a great hulk of a strong, warm, all-embracing guy in whose arms, under whose belly, you could dream of drowning. Many women seek the charms of heavyset men, men who are stout or portly, chubby or tubby, paunchy, pudgy, or plump, hulky, bulky, brawny and thick, strapping, imposing, substantial, a chunk.

Desperately poor people are undernourished; many working-class poor are fat. They pour their money into food and booze, and they find insulation in their fat against a scary world, where lack may at any moment brutally prevail. Their fat defends them against a cold wind, gives them bulk with which to feel stronger, and allows them to eliminate from their daily negotiations a great many desperate options.

Statisticians were amazed to discover what was everywhere visible, the jump in obesity from 1980 to 1991, when the percentage of adults who are overweight went abruptly from being a fourth to being a third of their number, according to the CDC.° The eighties also witnessed the steady impoverishment of the poor and middle class. You get fatter in this country as you get poorer, thinner as you get rich. The highest proportion of overweight people are black non-Hispanic women (49.5 percent) and Mexican-American women (47.9 percent). What you weigh has more to do with what's in your pocket than what's in your food. Oprah is probably genetically disposed to be fat, but her edifying example reveals that genetics is no fatality. In America money triumphs over the most resistant fat, which eventually recedes, finally suc-

° *New York Times,* July 17, 1994.

cumbing to the total regimes that only the rich or the fanatical can afford.

I think of my mother, who is beautiful and fat. Who is obese by the doctor's rule. She has lived an excellent life, the last forty years of which she has struggled to conform herself to the ideal of beauty that told her she had to be thin. And she did get thin, many times, at vast expense. She lost thousands of pounds of fat, and the more she lost the more she gained, and fat she is to the end. And I love her fat so much. I only wish there were more of it that I could love. I rage sometimes at the way she seems to have been manipulated by the ideal that the medical-health-beauty industry sells. But at other times, I recognize that she has never been complacently fat. She has provided herself with the most rigorous check on the pleasure she compulsively seeks. My mother goes to the supermarket to buy some frozen health dinners, grabs a Snickers bar at the cash register, and eats it on the way to the car. First she feels shame for having eaten all that (*obesus*). And then she forgets she ate it at all.

Dieting and overeating is a way of life for my mother; the nature of the quest, the rhythm it installs, is worthy of more respect than it normally receives. It is a kind of yoga, in which you give yourself the pleasure that you simultaneously sacrifice in the name of a higher ideal, making a ritual out of the dialectic of desire and its overcoming. Dieting while growing fatter is a kind of spiritual exercise. Every time you transgress that ideal, every time you break your resolutions and see the goal slip farther away, you feel such guilt and shame that you eat even more, for consolation and in defiance. More fat motivates more desperate diets, and the yo-yo builds mountains of it. The health industry has been stigmatizing fat for years, and people are fatter than ever. Obesity in girls has increased from 14 percent in 1981 to 24 percent, according to a recent Health Canada study. "A government survey found that the average weight of Americans 25 to 30 years old rose a whopping 10 pounds from 1985 to 1992, to 173 pounds for men and 148 pounds for women."° A lot of people blame TV: more watching of more commercials, like, for food, which brilliantly incite you to snack on the couch. Some people think, as I do, you also get fat just from watching television, not just from eating while you're watching, but from sitting there passively incorporating (absorbing/imbibing/ingesting) video into your body. Anyway, fat is back. McDonald's hottest item is its triple bacon cheeseburger.

If you need more proof, here it is, the most astounding news of all; they've recently revised significantly upward, yeah!, the ranges of ideal weight. I said "they"—I mean "Our Gods," statisticians in the bowels of the Center for Disease Control, actuaries behind gray partitions in Hartford, who (like Wallace Stevens in their way) divine the limits of the ideal. The U.S. Department of Agriculture, as always pushing food, has just issued new guidelines defining the "maximum desirable weight" for a man 6′ 2½″; newly revised, it turns out to be 210 pounds—exactly, as it happens, the weight at which Bill Clinton desirably weighed in at his last presidential checkup. In the race to accommodate more and more fat, one expert at Yale suggests that the best weight for most people is simply the lowest one they've been able to maintain for a year as an adult without struggling. Sound good?

It used to be that your ideal weight meant being painfully thin. I'm 5′ 8½″; my ideal weight is 142 pounds. At 142 pounds my

° *U.S. News and World Report,* May 16, 1994.

mother would begin to weep for me. So they changed ideal weight to desirable weight, in order to reflect the difference between fat before and fat after thirty-five. After thirty-five you are allowed to gain a half pound to a pound a year and still be in range. At my age and at my weight, that means I ought to weigh between 142 and 179 pounds. If I let myself accept that upper range as my maximum desirable weight, I could have a really good fat day. But who are we kidding? One look in the mirror at 179 pounds and I'm thinking liposuction.

At the same time, doctors, as ever faddish, cite new evidence that thin people die young. The Clinical Director of the National Institute on Aging observes that people middle-aged and older seem to live longer if they're "a bit on the pudgy side." Their fat nourishes them; reserves of it help them survive illnesses. In old age, it gives you strength and protection. That view and the conclusions drawn are hotly contested by the majority of professional people, dietitians and doctors who, viewing the issue dispassionately, insist that is wrong. They still encourage their patients, of all ages, to take drastic measures to reduce their risk of heart and other ailments that result, they believe, from unhealthy overweight. In the end, what is one to do?

Why are Americans obese? Ask a Frenchman. It's not the fat we eat. I mean I have friends from California who won't go to Paris because they might have to eat there, where everything is fat or prepared in fat. Vegetables are rare. The French hate green. Butter and cheese fill French veins, organ meats and goose fat load their tables; they eat much steak and fried potatoes, and dessert is ineluctable. And yet they remain as a people incomparably less obese than Americans. Ask a French woman, who knows America, why Americans are obese and she'll say, No discipline of eating. Despite inroads of fast food and progressive industrialization, French eating remains centered on rituals of the meal, with its disciplines. The first rule is no eating between meals. At the beginning of every meal the French wish each other *"Bon appétit."* Hunger, the desire to eat, is something to be wished, to be cultivated. Imagine wishing anyone hunger in America. The slightest hint of hunger here instantly provokes a rush to snack. Americans eat all day long, and food is everywhere available. You can eat anything, at any time, in any place between meals or at any meal. In France, you have to finish your cheese before you get dessert. Pleasure is not immediate; the meal installs an economy of pleasure, which again means manipulating hunger, holding off eating in order to eat later, with more pleasure and heightened discrimination.

Americans have bad eating habits. When desperately poor people eat the diet, say, of a German peasant they don't become obese; if they eat the same diet, in larger quantities, having become working-class poor, they get fat. To diminish obesity in this country you would have not to change diet, but to change habits. And to do that would represent an intolerable intrusion of government into our already overregulated lives. And furthermore it is not even imaginable, politically, that any institution in this country would take on the industries that have made vast fortunes exploiting and encouraging those habits. How would you get people to stop snacking in front of television—if you wanted to? You could make television interactively able to watch you and scold every time your hand goes to that bowl of peanuts. Big brother lies at the end of the dreams of some of those who want us, at all cost, to be healthy, slim, and beautiful. How do you change a society's habits? Try taking the candy bars away from the cash registers? Require bottlers to make smaller cans? Obesity is a price mankind pays for civilization. There's none of it in the jungle; there all fat is good. Domestic breeding produces fat animals, those who have been encouraged to eat more than they need to, for purposes of human need and pleasure. It's no accident, as Marxists used to say, that America, the richest nation, is the fattest. The more technological progress we achieve in creating comfort, the more obese we become. Machines that perform human functions much better than humans result in the progressive physical atrophy of the species. De-evolution contributes. We are, as Italo Svevo wrote, "the prosthetic" animal, the only creature who wears eyeglasses. Health, like the eyesight of the species, deteriorates as we become better able by means of machines and artificial substances to compensate for our growing enfeeblement. We are growing sicker and more unhealthy as civilization produces more garbage and toxins in order to fabricate the machines that give us the leisure to grow fatter and sicker. And in the meantime, we are being sold an increasingly distant ideal of desirable weight.

Part Two

THE THING

FAT

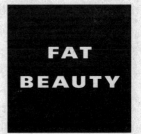

FAT BEAUTY

Suppose you wanted to find reasons to think that the current fashion in thin is due for a change. In a much disputed article, "Facing Food Scarcity," in a recent issue of *World Watch*° Lester R. Brown, the journal's publisher, trumpeted scary news of an estimate recently formed by the World Agricultural Outlook Board in Washington: "Measured in days of global consumption, the world's estimated carryover stocks of grain for 1996 had fallen to 49 days—the lowest level ever."† Carryover grain stocks are the key indicator of the world's capacity to meet the growing need for food. This cush-

° *World Watch,* October–November 1995, pp. 10–20.
† Ibid., pp. 10–11.

ion against scarcity is diminishing at this very moment. For example, China, in two years, has gone from being a net grain exporter to being a major importer, the grain-importing needs of Indonesia, Iran, Pakistan, Egypt, Ethiopia, Nigeria, Mexico, Bangladesh, and India have exploded, the global fish catch has begun to level off, if not decline. These latest developments reinforce the article's conclusion, stated in tones of dramatic alarm: "Indeed, for the first time in history, humanity is facing the prospect of a steady decline in both seafood and grain consumption per person for as far as we can see into the future."*

Under the present circumstances, in a world grown increasingly vulnerable, a sudden spell of drought worldwide could precipitate a food emergency. Its first effect, paradoxically, would be a drastic increase in the supply of food—of meat. Farmers everywhere would slaughter their animals rather than bear the expense of fattening them up with feed grown rare and precious. The oversupply would encourage people to gorge on meat, because it would suddenly be both very cheap and about to disappear from the tables of all but the rich. Thus, the poor, already fatter than the rich, would at first become even more fat, as a result of eating lots of cheap meat. But then, as meat vanished from their diet and scarcity spread, many would become thin, painfully thin. The rich, however, having despised fat when the poor were fat, would likely find, when the poor got thin, that fat was actually beautiful. It might happen almost overnight that the general perception of what is beautiful would all of a sudden change. Anna Nicole Smith would abruptly

---

* Ibid., p. 17.

appear on the cover of *Vogue*. Her generous forms have already made her the pinup model of a current generation of chubby chasers. But the future may be hers. She's shown she has a gift for timing, and I'd bet on her chances of being the next Betty Grable for the boys in Bosnia.

It wouldn't require a drastic lack of food—consider the oil shortage in the seventies—for the specter of scarcity to get our attention. Just the hint of a new global threat to the food supply might produce a decisive shift in the aesthetic appeal and nutritional value we attribute to fat. The first intimation of starvation on a worldwide scale might be enough to change the whole culture of food, heightening anxiety, investing fat with suddenly rediscovered benefits and unsuspected beauty.

There may be other reasons one could find to imagine that a change in taste will turn from thin to fat. But in truth no explanation may be possible or even necessary in order to understand what is bound to occur. Of one thing we can be sure: There will come a time, if civilization lasts, when fat again will be beautiful, and thin will be hated. Like most shifts in fashion, this one will dutifully obey the invisible, cyclical principle that seems to be at work in all history, but especially in the history of fashion. The only rule is this: What is out will be in, what's in out. The fashion principle commands—preprograms and guarantees—that over long periods of history the great pendulum swings between loving thin and loving fat.

I once rode in a car with Roland Barthes, the great French critic, from New Haven to Ithaca. I asked him in Binghamton what he thought it meant that the Beatles had made long hair suddenly fashionable. Was it a sign of the effeminization of men in the sixties, a culture shift toward a new androgyny? Was it a sign of a return to an earlier moment of Romanticism, when long hair was the unpruned expression of some higher, freer consciousness? I went on with possible interpretations of this drastic shift in taste. At the end, Barthes shrugged. He thought it wasn't any of these things. For him the shift was purely formal. Since short hair had been the rule before, in the fifties, the new rule required long hair in its place. The only significant meaning to be found here is the arbitrary one guaranteeing that short skirts will climb after long ones, that color will burst after beige and neutral tones, thin belts will thicken over time, and high heels follow pumps, as the moon does the sun. Fashion is not a natural thing, but it obeys its own inherent logic. Fashion follows its own law, so the shift to fat could happen for no reason, no good reason that anyone can tell. Maybe we'll just get tired of thin. Such a move will be resisted, of course, by the health-beauty-fitness industry; after all, it has a giant stake in thin. But when fat comes back, the industry will surely find other ways to make money out of people's anxieties. When fat returns, commentators will, after the fact, doubtless find compelling reasons to explain what occurred, why a sudden shift in taste. But the fashion swing, like a real one hung from a branch, obeys only the rule that says it must always swing in a direction opposite from where it's been.

To demonstrate this principle, I invite the reader on a quick little trip through the history of fat. Fat History is a subject that has only just begun to be written, although it has already produced two or three magnificent works. Hillel Schwartz and Roberta Reid, in particular, have enlarged our understanding of social attitudes in America toward fat—toward dieting and the regime of thin. I propose a more rapid and much more superficial survey of nothing less than the whole history of fat beauty, starting with cave women.

The first figures found that depict the human body are thought to be more than fifteen thousand years old; they are all female, all very round and bumpy, with erotic zones (tits, belly, ass) that protrude abundantly. These Venuses, for that's what archaeologists call these chubby little Stone Age statues—have been found in caves, especially in Germany and Italy but widely from France to Siberia.

The most famous of course is the Venus of Willendorf, a little figure four and a half inches tall, endowed with the most extraordinary proportions. Twenty thousand years ago, more or less, this magnificently abundant woman was carved out of soapstone, her enormous proportions compressed within a tiny compass. Projected to a life-size scale, she's about the fattest woman one can imagine. Two enormous mountains for breasts, perfectly rounded, plumped-up mounds, tower above her vast taut belly. While the hips curve into an endless ass, the giant thighs taper to thin legs cut off at the ankles. At the focus of all these immense sweeping hills of flesh is a fat and beautifully fashioned vulva. In the center of it all is a navel, vast and dark and deep.

Venuses, we know, are goddesses of love, but archaeologists don't get it. With their professional bias in favor of use and usefulness, they assume these figures must be fertility fetishes, serving some ritual purposes—objects of prayer fashioned to foster conception and protect pregnancy. They make that assumption based on the further assumption that since all of these figures are fat—fat

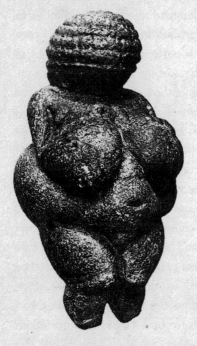

Venus of Willendorf

breasts and bellies and thighs—they must be pregnant. To be sure, there is some direct proportion between the amount of fat a woman bears and her capacity to bear children. Fat is fertile; we have already pointed that out. Certainly, we know that the obverse is even more likely to be the case: thin women are less fertile, less successful at bearing children. After a certain point of emaciation, menstruation stops altogether, and fertility vanishes. The advantages of fat were surely even more pressing to our ancestors in the cave; when famine lurked as a constant menace, a pregnant mother blessed her fat's insurance against the loss of her future child.

But the question remains. What certainty do we have that these are ritual objects, magical amulets, or voodoo dolls? How do we know that their shapes and form are intended to cause the condition they seem to represent? Why do they have to be useful? Scientists, who aren't supposed to take beauty into account, assume that cave people were not able to distinguish their love of what was beautiful from their desire to replenish the supply of human workers. But when you look at these amazing figures in three dimensions, in the very round, you see a lot of things sticking out on every side. Asses are no less the focus of artistic attention than breasts or vast, prominent bellies, and that's important. In humans who face each other in love, asses came to have to do more with pleasure than with reproduction, and one that sticks out behind, with the same assertive audacity as bubble breasts in front, is hot. A fat ass doesn't serve any reproductive function. Except that it's fat, and in general fat is fertile. A big beautiful ass on these figures is an object of admiration and a spur to dreaming, a sort of pillow on which our grottoed ancestors may well have fantasized fat, and in times of scarcity dreamt of its pleasures. In the dreams of the caveman, these goddesses gambol at play in fat fields and splash in lively streams, lovely ladies abounding in the lush landscapes that compose his visions of paradise.

Nothing prevents us from assuming that these statues were absolutely useless, were simply beautiful—like more recent Venuses, mere representations of ideal feminine beauty. I believe it when I look at another soapstone figure from the Balzi Rossi cave, in Ventimiglia, on the border of what is now France and Italy. Right there, at the heart of what we now know as the Riviera, they found this lit-

tle figure of a Stone Age bathing beauty with Bardot proportions—
with tits and ass that stir the mind like a swelling Ode to Joy or La
Marseillaise. And in between, you notice, she has the flattest stomach, a flat expanse of firmed-up waist stretching between the ballooning boobs on top and the rest. This woman is not pregnant.

She has a waist. Since no other animal in nature has a waist, one
could say that it distinguishes humans from animals. Humans alone
are moved by the erotic power of the shapely curves that narrow at
the waist and open to embrace the hips and breasts. Formally
speaking, the waist lends to the shape of the body its dynamic asymmetry. It permits the body to be seen not as a single block but as a
balanced arrangement of distinctly different blocks—the flat broad
plain of the chest or the globes of breasts and the triangle between
them are in a certain relation of symmetry or asymmetry with the
oval of the stomach or the sturdy rectangle of a muscular torso.
Since the ancient Greeks, sculptors have exploited the pose that
consists in putting your weight on one foot. The French have a
name for it, *déhanchement;* it means swinging, or twisting, or sticking out a hip. The vital, mobile beauty of Greek statues, compared
to Egyptian ones, depends in part on the way the Greek pose
breaks the straight-on symmetry of the body, and turns it into a
moving architecture of thrusts and counterthrusts, concavities and
convexities, which multiply the curves that the waist initiates.

The fact that the Balzi Rossi figure has a waist doesn't exclude,
I suppose, the possibility that it represents fertility. But I think it's
just as plausible to think it was primarily an object of erotic and sensual pleasure. Maybe the sculptor just loved the business of chisel-
ing out of soft, yielding stone the voluminous bodies of beautiful fat

women. Perhaps he enjoyed rubbing the curves of her breasts until the stone yielded the high gloss of the perfectly rounded forms. This may be the first example of the sort of art that today would arouse the wrath of censors—art designed with a view to exciting aroused attention. These objects may be pure pornography, lascivious shapes of the sculptor's erotic fantasy, made to be scoped and fondled, but only with one hand. Why shouldn't their fat be a sign of exuberant sex? After all, there are African tribes that seclude their brides before marriage, in order to fatten them up, and certain Polynesian tribes have great reverence for women who reach two hundred or three hundred pounds.[*]

But I rest my case on the Venus of Laussel, found in a cave in Dordogne. The proportions have acquired a degree of fat realism that's quite astonishing. This lady has no waist. But she has curves, rolls and rolls of multiplying layers of fat, ballooning into thighs, and hips, and ample pendulous breasts. Delicate fingers are spread out across the belly, perhaps patting, perhaps pointing to the riches contained within and below. The head is turned as if to suck on what the lady in her other hand is holding, what art historians delicately call the horn of a bull. If there are times when a horn is only a horn, and not a phallus, this one should be considered a horn of plenty, the first cornucopia in art—an emblem of the profusion of nature and a sign for the generosity of women's bodies.

Throughout the Middle Ages, women, especially fat ones, have been identified with the figure of *copia,* with the idea of plentiful

[*] Roberta Pollack Seid, *Never Too Thin: Why Women Are at War with Their Bodies* (New York: Prentice Hall, 1989), p. 45.

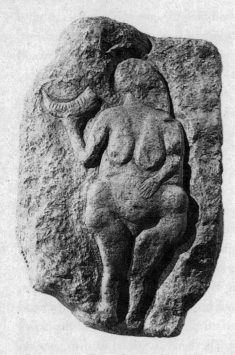

Venus of Laussel

abundance. As we have seen, that overflowing abundance has also for a long time been associated with the propensity of women to talk excessively. Maybe that's why the Venus of Laussel, head turned to drink or blow, could just as well be seen, anachronistically, to be speaking on the horn.

If you look at the Venus of Laussel and compare her to Nefertiti, the fabulous beauty of ancient Egypt, you get some sense of the vast cycles of fat and thin that punctuate human history. Ten or fifteen thousand years after the Stone Age Venus, in the time of Anket-Amon, lived the most beautiful woman in antiquity, Nefertiti, the mother of Tutankhamen. Her son, despite having died young, is today the most famous pharaoh, lucky that his tomb was found immaculately untouched by grave robbers. Nefertiti's body bears only the most distant relation to the ideal of Stone Age beauty. The elegance of her lines, compared to the behemoth in soapstone, is still very far from suggesting anything like the bony angular thinness we have lately come to love. She is no Kate Moss. The breasts are beautiful but, in proportion to the hips, small. The belly is ample and only slightly protuberant, but the thighs are solid and embracing.

The famous head of Nefertiti displays the incomparable thinness and angular tilt of her neck, and the barest trace of a smile. The graceful elegance of the head is accentuated by the slender crown she wore, one that extends the line of the nape and resembles no other crown worn by Egyptian queens. Not only beautiful but chic, she knew what looks good. But what makes her face so immediately recognizable, the source of its extraordinary fascination, is the thin upbeat line of the smile that permanently seems to play at the corners of her exquisite lips. Those lips are more than features of her beauty; they hint at moods that on her face look witty, sharply intelligent, often amused. Nefertiti's beauty is often called immortal. What's immortal, it seems to me, is the slender elegance of her neck and the mystery of that smile. I still can't believe how perfectly her mouth resembles that of Claudia Schiffer, whose greatest charm, above the neck, abides in the gentle upturned corners of her mouth that lend that face its breath-stopping look of sweet or sexy amusement. Cover her face, all but her mouth, and Claudia, like Nefertiti, is instantly recognizable.

Her facial resemblance to the queen of Egypt can't obscure the difference between their bodies. Compared to the Venus of Willendorf, both these ladies may be thought to be thin. But, comparing idealized statues and airbrushed photos, Claudia Schiffer, the modern model, is skinny compared to Nefertiti, despite having much larger breasts. (Skinny as she is, Claudia is often cited as one of the few voluptuous top models who don't look utterly anorexic.) The shape and widths of Claudia Schiffer's body correspond to the peculiar ideal of beauty invented in our century, the one that wants women to be (or seem to be) larger around the breasts than around the hips. Compare her to Nefertiti, whose hips and thighs swell from the waist, whose stomach protrudes in two gentle mounds. The stomach of Claudia Schiffer (you could almost call it an ab) is alarmingly flat. In the photos taken by Karl Lagerfeld of Claudia barely dressed, her stomach has the emaciated flatness of one that has been tightened and toned, stretched and loosened by years of exercise and yo-yo dieting—the price her beauty pays to the anorexic ideal of designers. Compared to the beauty of antiquity or classical times, the elongated shape of Claudia's body lacks the solid form and weighty movement that lend authority and dignity to a royal body.

Of course, too much fatness promotes stolid symmetry, at the expense of more fluid, plastic qualities permitted by thin: imbalance, precariousness, complication of line. It's hard to sculpt fat wrestlers, for example. Kenneth Clark, with his classical taste, understood that the beauty of the nude body required both symmetry and asymmetry in the right places, both fat and thin, neither wholly one nor entirely the other.

You mustn't be too thin or too fat, thought the ancient Greeks. In his book *The Nude*, Clark gives us a figured vase from the fifth century B.C., on which four men are drawn.* On one side of the jar are two hunky athletes, throwing the discus and javelin; they are muscular, solid, and lithe. On the other side, clearly separated from the action, is a fat young man seen in profile, with a big belly, turning his back to the games. Next to him is a skinny guy, facing the athletes but seeming to pull away as far as he can from the action. The moral of the jar seems unambiguous: both fat and thin are at odds with the Greek ideal of vigorous male beauty. Greeks, then as now, loved their fat. Homer is full of roasting meat. At the same time, we know that the Spartans exiled a citizen for being too fat. A fat body for the Greeks lacked the asymmetry of lithe, moving lines that belong to the restless energy of thin. But thin, similarly for them, lacked the noble thickness that lends dignity and a commanding air to those perfect bodies, to these embodiments of the very gods themselves.

The Greeks, as in all things, took a moderate position toward fat, and aspired to a golden mean. The only fat Greek statues are those of *sileni*, satyrs, half man and half goat, related to Bacchus, the god of wine and festivity. Greek women reputedly envied the wasp waist of Etruscan women, who, it was believed, "had found a magic potion that kept them slim."* Hippocrates, the father of Greek medicine, considered fat a disease. And Socrates danced every morning as a way of controlling his weight. Dancing every

---

* Kenneth Clark, *The Nude: A Study in Ideal Form* (Princeton, N.J.: Princeton University Press, 1956).

morning is a form of dieting little practiced in the world today, but one that ought perhaps to be revived. Philosophical dieting. Maybe Richard Simmons is right; the only way you can truly stay thin is by dancing every day, because if it doesn't work, it doesn't matter. You will have danced every day of your life. Unless you don't think that what Richard Simmons is doing is dancing.

Aphrodite by our standards is fat. If you take another look at the Venus de Milo, you have to be impressed by her girth. She's a chunk—immense round hips, great tits, this is a big girl! Her beauty lies in the proportions of her body, not in its slenderness. She's not chic, like Nefertiti, she doesn't immediately arouse you with some mysterious electric spark—like what flies from the corner of Claudia's mouth, or from the jut of a bony hip, or from the racy elongated curves of these strange and exciting poses. But Venus de Milo is beautiful, with an antique beauty that touches a viewer more profoundly. Her thickness is "fruitful and robust," says Kenneth Clark and, compared to more conventional nudes, she rises up, he says, "like an elm tree in a field of corn."* She is both vigorous and fat, with no skinny chest, but a vast expanse of her neck and shoulders and breasts. It is no wonder that less than one hundred years ago we admired the compelling spectacle of abundant jewels flashing around the neck of a beautiful woman dressed in a gown from which poured the full extent of her magnificent chest.

There are Etruscan tombs known as the Obesii, which depict the deceased male lying on top of his sarcophagus, half draped, resting on one arm, with his great big gut hanging out. The Romans

* Seid, p. 46.

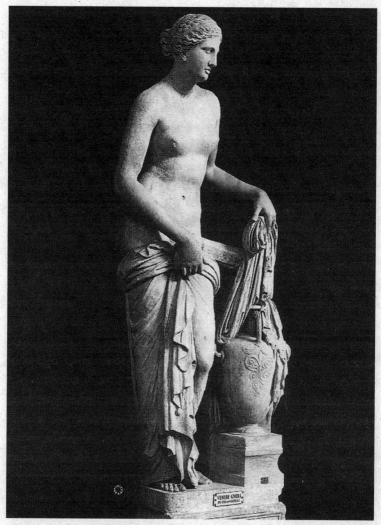

Aphrodite of Cnidus, after Praxiteles

used to make fun of the fat Etruscans, but the statues make you think that those stomachs had some sort of social significance, a sign of the departed's once substantial role in the city. Kenneth Clark thinks the Etruscan sculptors were just good realists, who were accurately depicting the look of middle-aged men, half naked, lying down.

In Roman times, the cult of the body was displaced by preoccupations with dress and adornment. Clothing concealed the body and lent it the dignity that Roman bodies might lack. The Romans weren't as athletic as the Greeks; their tastes went in more for banqueting. The *vomitorium* to which Romans retired in the midst of banquets was devised, it seems, less to prevent fat than to encourage more eating. Remember that Nero was fat.

To be sure, there is some evidence of the surgical removal of fat in Roman and Byzantine times. The fantasy of liposuction has roots that go very deep in our culture. Fat has always been conceived as a kind of cancerous growth, inessential to the body or its image, an excrescence, a corruption of the flesh whose removal left the body intact and in better shape. Fat is something that we wear; it is on the outside of our inside. It doesn't belong to us exactly, and it doesn't belong where we find it. We dream of its being removed from us, leaving our essential being not only unaffected and unchanged but more purely, because more thinly, itself. For the Greeks and Romans, fat in moderation was a principal source of pleasure and a major component of beauty.

Kenneth Clark, in *The Nude*, begins by observing that many civilizations have no art of the nude. Consider the Orient, where neither in Japan or China or elsewhere is there a long and ancient tradition of representing beautiful naked bodies. It is first in the West, and with the culture of the Greeks, that the naked body becomes a nude, the object of artistic contemplation and representation. The greatness of Clark's book, as a piece of art history, lies in the way he shows the two basic models of the body on which the whole art of the nude has been based. There's the classical nude and the Gothic. The difference, we might say, is a question of fat in the right or wrong places.

According to Kenneth Clark, with the triumph of Christianity over paganism, "the body ceased to be a mirror of divine perfection and became an object of humiliation and shame."[*] Whereas the Greeks wanted to celebrate the athlete's nobility in the gym, the earliest medieval statues of humans undressed represent the shame and humiliation of Adam and Eve. After the Fall, scales fell from their eyes and they perceived that they were not nude, but naked as peeled shrimp. The pious Christian ideal of beauty starts there, in the humiliation of the flesh. It bespeaks a hatred of every fleshy thing that prevents the soul from instantly achieving its spiritual destiny. Flesh was no longer the blessed stuff in which the gods became present among humans. The beauty of its forms was censored by Judeo-Christian taboos surrounding graven images, and its seductions were demonized by Christian morals. The landscape of the human body was no longer deemed to enact the mysteries of creation, proposing to the eye of the dazzled spectator an incomparable vision of tension and ease, force and yielding, strength and softness. In the Gothic period, the body was often angular, sharp, and mean.

[*] Clark, p. 309.

Its gauntness was evidence of the mortification of the flesh, punished for its power to entice the soul toward pleasure, away from grace. Whereas for the pagan Greeks the body was the place where physical pleasure and divine grace intermingled harmoniously, Judaism despised the body for its impurities and required its constant ritual purification. Christian teaching preached that pagan statues of Greek and Roman gods, under their beautiful guises, were actually devils, little demons that tempted thoughts away from the path of Christ. In early Christian times, one aspired not to the body of the athlete but to the anorexic skeleton of the anchorite, or hermit, who retreated from the material world, from all its delicious pleasures. For Christians, appetite is a lure that ensnares the soul and perverts its pious impulses. Finally, in Islam, the body becomes the site for harsh rituals of self-abnegation. Shiite Muslims parade through the streets on occasion flagellating themselves with cruel metal whips until blood flows.

Schiller, in *The Aesthetic Education,* argued that Greeks burned their dead because they aspired to what they lacked—a fully grasped understanding of the eternal infinite possessed by Judeo-Christianity. By contrast, Christians and Jews bury their dead, because they aspire to what the Greeks lack: a fully realized, pagan sense of the immediate, incarnated presence of divinity in the flesh.

Even today, one cannot help believing that the current fashion for thin is linked to an upsurge of pious belief. Fat, like a Greek god, has become a devil. Throughout most of human history, fat has been thought to be the best thing, the most beautiful and desirable stuff of all. But at certain moments, in periods of high religious sentiment, fat comes to be despised. For the early Christians, for the medieval Gothic period, during the period of Romanticism, fat was taken as the emblem of all the mortal weight of sin arising from temptations to which the flesh is given. The Gothic idea or ideal of the pious body was ethereal—gaunt, bony, and potbellied.

Why was the Gothic belly a pot? In the earliest representations of Eve, leaving the Garden of Eden, she is engraved with skinny legs, small breasts, a long curving stomach. It's probably too simple to assume that her fat belly was supposed to be seen to be the pregnant destiny of Christian womanhood. This young lady isn't pregnant yet, but the rounded curve of her belly means that babies are on her horizon.

Just as we've seen with Stone Age figures, this pregnant interpretation of the Gothic belly may fail to account for what, after all, is simply a matter of taste. Compared to the Classical ideal, Kenneth Clark calls the Gothic body rarefied, because of the way it flattens the thrusting arc of the hip. Central to the body of the Greek and Roman nude was the "sensuous arc" formed by the hip and waist, which resulted from the figure being posed with its weight unevenly distributed, resting heavily on one foot.* The sexy arc formed by the jutting hip and flaring torso has the power to move us in ways that aren't rarefied at all. In ways that may be biological.

Texas professor Devendra Singh, you remember, believes the secret of sex appeal lies at the waist—or, to be precise, the waist-hip ratio calculated by dividing the waist measurement by the hip size. The smaller the waist in relation to the hip, the more desirable a

---

* Ibid., p. 315.

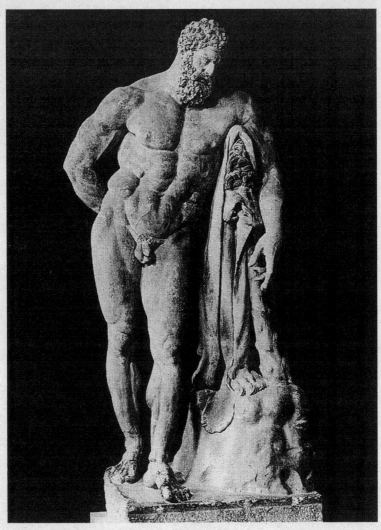

Farnese Hercules

woman is seen to be. As a result of her recent study, she concludes, "The waist is one of the distinguishing human features, such as speech, making tools and a sense of humor." "No other primate has one. We developed it as a result of another unique feature—standing upright. We needed bigger buttock muscles for walking on two legs."* A fat ass makes us human.

The Classical nude, both male and female, exploits the architectural and erotic possibilities of that breathtaking curve at buttocks and hip. But the Gothic nude tends to elongate the body, both male and female. In the Renaissance, the male body reasserts the Classical prerogatives, only it looks thicker. Thick is fat, as in German, the word *Dieck* means both. Thickness in men around the chest and waist still exerts a powerful attraction on women, and other men. Here's one version of that:

> He was naked. He stood there, the hair over his cock and balls emphasized by my own lack of covering. I was overcome by the sight of him. The chest, the full muscled stomach, the arms promising such strength. Mr. Benson, my master, my man, the one for whom I would do anything.[†]

That's how John Preston's narrator, a submissive slave to S/M, describes the moment when he sees his master undressed. What rivets his attention to the body of the male master is the fullness and strength of the torso. Not the arc but the thickness of the chest and

---

* *Irish Times,* November 10, 1994.
[†] John Preston, *Mr. Benson.* (New York: Bad Boy Press, 1992), p. 91.

stomach—the density of the muscled flesh is what the naked slave loves. Just like Michelangelo. Look at the great allegorical statues of Day or Dawn, or consider the series called Captives, or think of some of the male figures in *The Last Judgment,* there you'll see Michelangelo thickening the stomachs on these heroic guys almost to the point of becoming obese and funny. But for him, the whole drama and pathos of what he was trying to express, in these heroic drawings and carvings in stone, writhed into life in the thick intensity of muscle and fat at the shoulder and chest and waist. It's true that Michelangelo liked lithe boys like his *David*—slim waisted, with bony ribs. But as he aged he painted more and more obsessively those thick waists on females as well as males. His late statues of women, sculpted for the pope's tomb, look like men lying down wearing oranges on their chest. But Michelangelo was less interested in the difference between male and female than in that between master and slave. He must have loved slaves dearly, because he made so many of them, but his slaves, powerful, rippling bodies, serve to represent the mystery of thick flesh—its humbling power to move us profoundly. The flesh to which we wish to submit is thick and heavy and tragic.

In France, in the sixteenth century, the first great attempts to represent naked beauty since the Dark Ages gave rise to the School of Fontainebleau. Mannerist artists brought from Italy to France by Francis I infused the moving, dynamic lines of the South with severe Gothic angularity to produce strangely disturbing, extravagantly elegant elongated nudes. Kenneth Clark observes that the legs of Cellini's *Nymph of Fontainebleau* are six times the length of her head, compared to the Classical model, which dictated three.

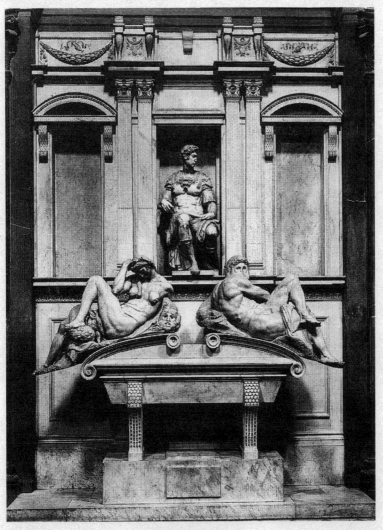

Michelangelo's tomb

These figures, with their "somewhat ridiculous shape—feet and hands too fine for honest work, bodies too thin for childbearing, and heads too small to contain a single thought," says Clark, are the embodiment of chic. The beauty they embody is antinatural; they bear no relation to real women, but only to impossible ideas of women, whose illusion they create. Clark writes, "The goddess of mannerism is the eternal feminine of the fashion plate."[*] Top models, with their emaciated forms, vacant stares, and otherworldly airs are the latest embodiment of mannerist chic, the most persistent incarnations of the insubstantial Gothic ideal.

Clark is aware that this antinatural vision of chic has its victories in the history of art. It has triumphed in the twentieth century. But we should not be deluded, he tells us, into thinking that the beauty that's in fashion is the only form of it or the greatest. As he says, when we are in need of "greater nourishment," the lover of beauty cannot be satisfied with the amusing or provocative detours of chichi, the strange thin forms that unreal beauty takes. When a connoisseur of Venus *naturalis* wants to drink deeply of the springs of feminine beauty and consume with eyes the most substantial fruits of flesh, it is to Rubens he must turn. Clark writes, "The golden hair and swelling bosoms of his *Graces* are hymns of thanksgiving for abundance, and they are placed before us with the same unselfconscious piety as the sheaves of corn and piled-up pumpkins that decorate a village church at harvest festival."[†] These women are cornucopia, with bodies that swell and plump. The graces hold and

[*] Clark, p. 139.
[†] Ibid., p. 140.

squeeze each other's arms, as if even they cannot get enough of their exuberant fleshy beauty. Rubens was attracted by the twist and sweep, by the large arc of a hip, and "the shining expanse of . . . stomach."* He loves the comprehensiveness of these bodies, the way they sweep the eye around with arcs and twists, intriguing rolls and blushing dimples. The roundness of these fat women inspires in the onlooker an enormously powerful desire to embrace them, to be embraced in their enclosing perfumed thicket of flesh.

You have to love the sweetness of these faces, the transparent delicacy of the palest skin, and the way these ladies seem to float and dance like exuberant pillows, billowing flesh enchanting the viewer with a spectacle of boundless grace, when nature in its abundance seems perfectly attuned to fostering the happiness of humanity.

In the seventeenth century, at the dawn of classical rationality, one could still believe in the harmony of a rational natural order with a deeply felt divine plan. For Rubens, there was no contradiction between reason and faith. The world was good and God-given, and humanity through its own rational powers could understand nature and improve it. Clark repeatedly refers to the sweetness and generosity of Rubens's fat women—qualities very far removed from the hard, angular principles of chic.

Kenneth Clark likes painters who like fat girls. To be sure, he dismisses the Venus of Willendorf. She is fatness, he thinks, grown to be a mere symbol of fertility. He has little interest in the sexy mounds of the statuette, carved so softly in stone. It's enough that the fat be fertile to turn Sir Kenneth off. When it comes to really

---

* Ibid., p. 144.

fat, he backs away from his otherwise acutely trained sense of the beauty of what is solid, substantial, what has density and aplomb— the quality of being well centered and perfectly balanced. For him, her fat is too fat.

But there are other forms of fat he defends indignantly. Kenneth Clark asks the reader and himself, "Why do we burn with indignation when we hear people who believe themselves to have good taste dismissing Rubens as a painter of fat naked women and even applying the epithet 'vulgar'?"* Why does he burn when he hears that? Because these people, who are supposed to have taste, are the most tasteless of all. These are people so concerned with chic that they cannot see beauty; they consider fat vulgar and thereby reveal the vulgarity of their taste. Clark, more refined than these vulgarians who think fat is vulgar, has taste, appreciates the taste of fat. Fat makes Rubens's nude one of the highest summits of the art of the nude in all of history.

"Rubens," Clark says, "wished his figures to have weight. So did the men of the Renaissance, and they sought to achieve it by closed forms, which had the ideal solidity of the sphere or the cylinder."† The forms of fat women are closed forms, and they evoke the desire to enclose them, to comprehend their sweeping arms in the sweep of our arms. The women of Rubens give rise to the desire to sweep them up, to feel their weight and solidity, to give oneself the incredible sweetness of their all-embracing fat. Clark gives us in *The Nude* the picture by Rubens entitled *The Rape of the Two Daughters of*

---

* Ibid., p. 139.
† Ibid., p. 144.

Leukippos. Rape may be understood here in its first sense, which is that of seizing hold of, from Latin *rapere,* grasping, comprehending. You could imagine this painting to be a sort of allegory of the Classical period, in which male reason surrounds, seizes upon, grasps, and comprehends an idea of feminine solidity. This idea of the fat woman is both intellectual and erotic—an image of ideal beauty in which what is most sensual is linked to what is most comprehensive, universal—the ennobling mixture of voluminous flesh with a transcendent idea of immensity. A single, glistening cylinder of fat, this luscious fat girl stands for all that the rational mind and the love of beauty desire to possess, to surround and carry off—the whole weight and wealth of human nature. The body of a Rubens' woman is, according to Clark, "plump and pearly."[*]

Rubens did for the female nude what Michelangelo had already done for the male. Both great artists discovered whole new levels of expressivity in the form of the human body by imagining it thick or plump. Michelangelo's figures suffer (or profit) from what Clark calls "the peculiar thickening of the torso (increased, even, in correction)."[†] This means that as Michelangelo worked and reworked his drawings of male nudes, he tended more and more to broaden the torso, to give it ever wider girth, more ample expanse of fat and muscle. Some figures, like the Christ of *The Last Judgment,* look almost misshapen, from the chest down. But they nevertheless attain, in Clark's eyes, "a Pheidian splendor." Like Pheidias, the greatest sculptor in ancient Greece, Michaelangelo

[*] Ibid., p. 148.
[†] Ibid., p. 60.

not only reproduces the beauty of gods, he infuses his heroic images with a palpable aura, a pearly sign of the presence of divinity in the flesh. Great artists find their gods incarnate, embodied in the beauty of amply proportioned fat.

With the Christian Middle Ages, moral attitudes toward flesh reversed the classical model of beauty. The body as the locus of pleasure and hence of sin was depreciated and emaciation became a sign of spiritual elevation—of turning away from the fleshpots of this world. Think of the Venus de Milo, then think of the poor bodies of those emaciated, saintly, self-denying women, mostly nuns, who have been called, by Rudolph Bell, "holy anorexics." The first nude figures one sees in medieval art are Adam and Eve, whose nakedness is an occasion, not for celebration, but for shame and self-concealment. The Gothic woman, as she is represented in statues and images, displays a body shape and structure fundamentally different from the female body admired in Classical Antiquity. Of the Gothic woman, Clark says, "Her pelvis is wider, her chest narrower, her waist higher; above all, there is the prominence given to her stomach."° The hint of fertility is the only exception permitted to the general thinning and elongation of the female form. The woman's body is no longer seen and loved for itself, as an object of sensual contemplation, but envisaged as a vessel devoted to reproduction. The thinness of these Gothic bodies, which have their own mannered charm, negotiates a compromise between the allure of flesh and the rigors of spirit. On the one hand, there's the old urge to look hard at the body in order to paint or sculpt it, and, on the

° Ibid., p. 317.

other, the church's taboo on undressed flesh. Countering the pure, pagan pleasure of eyeing gorgeous flesh, the Gothic skinny is a philosophical decision and a moral judgment about the place of the body in the hierarchy of values.

The emaciated Gothic ideal was not generally shared by the lower classes in the Middle Ages and Renaissance. Kristoff Glamann, quoted in Mennell, argues that as far as they were concerned, eating made you handsome. A thin wife brought disgrace to a peasant, but of a plump one it was said that "a man will love her and not begrudge the food she eats" [Mennell 30]. Men, too, were supposed to be stout, to judge, say, from the painter Breughel's scenes of high life and low, where mostly everyone is tubby, afloat in rolling fat, while gluttony abounds.

In the sixteenth and seventeenth centuries, gluttony was widespread, even at the highest levels of society. Catherine de Médicis was known for her enormous appetite and frequent dyspepsia. Henry VIII was gargantuan in his appetite. Gargantua, the royal giant invented by Rabelais, as an infant drank the milk of 17,913 cows, and counted eighteen adipose chins.° In the seventheenth century, at Versailles, Louis XIV consumed prodigious amounts of food and became lustrously, heroically fat. At his court, the Princess Palatine died from overeating.

The eighteenth century represented a movement away from overeating toward greater refinement of taste, as cuisines became more delicate and taste more subtle. But even thin was not so

° Hillel Schwartz, *Never Satisfied: A Cultural History of Diets, Fantasies, and Fat.* (New York: Free Press, 1986), p. 9.

skinny back then, by our current standards: Madame de Pompadour—111 pounds and only 5'1" tall—complained of being emaciated. Louis XVI was the exception that confirmed the rule.* His morbid obesity became an emblem of an aristocratic class grown bloated with self-satisfaction, inert from conservatism, and, like Louis himself, hugely impotent. He was so fat, it is said, he could not see his penis. Louis was already a scandal on his wedding day, when he so incapacitated himself with food and drink, that his grandfather, Louis XV, then the king, expressed outrage and muttered foreboding about the future of his dynasty. On his way to the guillotine, Louis asked for a little something to eat.

The hollow decadence of the old regime is often diagnosed in the taste it displayed, at the end of the eighteenth century, for frivolous flesh that seems gratuitous, floating on buttocks and bosoms in paintings by Watteau and Boucher. Fat is dimpled, all pink and fluffy in Boucher, the eighteenth century Rococo court painter. The creamy skin of those large dollops of pink women—ladies, really, with beautiful aristocratic faces, winsome, and proud—arouses hunger, quenches thirsts. They are at play on billowy couches, and the light suffusing their bodies illuminates the round pillows of downy linen and their satiny flesh, ballooning, effervescent, like bubbles of fat. They are dressed alluringly in the gauziest veils, which barely cover them—just enough to excite the wish to see what is plainly visible through the filmy, flimsy cloth. The most famous Boucher painting, in the Louvre, features a woman lying on her stomach with her ass in the air looking back in laughter at the

---

* Seid, p. 56.

painter. The gorgeous display of her colossal adiposity, her thundering, moonfaced, creviced posterior, evokes a vastly delicious, (sub)lunar landscape in which an explorer could lose himself in pleasure forever. O blessed fat!

The chunky butts on women in Boucher are full of fat. They remind us how beautifully it accumulates in places of particular erotic attention. The fat of a breast, the heft and weight of that fat that surrounds a beautifully formed nipple—the shape and roundness of that fat invites fondling. It calls out for touching. Butts lend themselves to be grabbed—that is, to be held in big handfuls and to

Turkish Bath *by Ingres*

be squeezed. Squeezing the fat on butts is for many people, men and women, the source of the most intense erotic pleasure. Only humans have fatty breasts. There are those like Desmond Morris who say that breasts are behinds, that in humans the breast is surrounded by fat to remind men of behinds, which they used to love when we went on all fours.

When a fat king is overthrown, the new republic loves thin. In the nineteenth century, post-revolutionary Europe was swept by the Romantic movement, a new conception of the relation of mind to body and with it an altered sense of what is beautiful—a new figure of fashion. Hamlet ceased to be played by fat actors; only those who were thin could look brooding and melancholic. The Romantic soul inhabits a slender body, one whose shape bespeaks a disinterested, ascetic relation to food and to the material world in general. The Romantic movement re-invented a Gothic ideal of thin, ethereal beauty, in order to evoke the idea of some edifying elevation beyond the flesh. Beauty, as it were, is removed from this world, freed from the inertia and impenetrability of this too too solid flesh. The world, in a Romantic perspective, is seen at a distance, as if from a rugged mountain top where bodies like spirits appear almost transparent—like clouds reflected in an Alpine lake. Being without the earth means to be un-fat. A sublime aesthetic, a taste for the sublime, replaced its eighteenth century opposite, the frivolous excess, the ornamental abundance of Rococo. Between 1800 and 1850, for the first time in almost four hundred years the look of thin once more looked beautiful. The French writer, Théophile Gautier, recalled that, during this period, when he was young, he could not have "accepted as a lyric poet anyone weighing more than 99 pounds."[*] Roberta Seid also notes that it was in 1832, at the height of the Romantic movement in Europe, that ballerinas first began dancing on point. The aspiration of the human body to approximate the human soul took form and body in these altered ideals of femininity. Even when fashion changed, around the 1850s, when both men and women began reverting to a heavier model, fat was still associated, not with gravity but with bubbly buoyancy.

By the end of the century, as we have seen, the Gay Nineties had brought the industrial world unprecedented wealth, and all classes aspired to look and feel fat. Men cultivated their corporations, and women squeezed their flesh in the middle with whale bone and leather in order to produce at both ends cascading avoirdupois. The exuberance of fat, its imposing assertiveness, its unfolding promise of ever more abundance sweeps everything before it until the first decade of the twentieth century, when, as if overnight, thin looked sleek and modern.

Until this century no one has ever dreamed of living in a skinny land. Fat has always been the shape of Utopia. Now, of course, the prejudice against fat seems universal and eternal; and thin belongs to what is truly good and beautiful. Nevertheless, there are those, even today, who dream of a fat utopia, and have written earnestly and vigorously in its favor. None has done so more eloquently than Hillel Schwartz. As he modestly asserts, at the end of his great book *Never Satisfied:* "No single critic has launched such an attack on dieting as I have launched here."[†] In a chapter entitled "Fat and

[*] Seid, p. 94.
[†] Schwartz, p. 332.

Happy," Schwartz describes the conditions that would thrive in "The Fat Society: A Utopia," in which fatness would be both admired and rewarded. Here are some of the rewards and pleasures that would accompany this utopia of fat:

1. Dinners would be "scrumptious, sociable, and warm."

2. Children would acquire no eating disorders because "feeding would be calm and loving, always sufficient, never forced."

3. Fat people would love their bodies and "dress expressively." Women, in particular, "would wear their weight with new conviction."

4. "A fat society would be a comforting society, less harried, more caring."

5. A fat society would be less harshly competitive, less devouring.°

Schwartz is one of the first, and certainly the most eloquent, to find in fat the emblem of Capitalism, a metaphor and index of our society's relation to consumption. We are all consumers, and the fat that we wear or the fat that we flee expresses a certain relation we have, as consumers, to the objects of our desire. Schwartz is one of those who has most carefully and thoroughly distinguished hunger from appetite. Hunger is a drive, a biological need motivated from within by the body's lack of what it needs; appetite is a desire, stimulated by the attraction or seduction of things outside the self that provoke an interest or inclination to eat. One's appetite can be stimulated, even if one is not hungry. Indeed, for some, that is the function of good cooking.

° Ibid.

According to Schwartz, the logic of capitalism, particularly in its late stages, expresses itself in the novel forms of dieting. On the surface, he argues, it might seem paradoxical to identify dieting and capitalism. After all, the capitalist is a consumer, a seeker after the commodities that excite his appetite. Dieting would seem to imply the opposite of consuming, and hence a form of resistance to the capitalist mode. The paradox would be a real one, a true antinomy, if dieting in fact succeeded for the most part in accomplishing what it aims to achieve. But writing in 1986, Schwartz can already feel confident about asserting as fact what has become massively evident in the meantime: diets don't work. Never have; never will. And it is precisely that fact that makes dieting such a perfect vehicle for launching a critique of capitalism. Dieters in truth, argues Schwartz, consume not less but more. "The diet is the supreme form for manipulating desire precisely because it is so frustrating."* Since capitalism depends on consumers consuming, the more they diet the more they frustrate desire, thereby magnifying its imperious demands. More diet means more appetite, and more appetite means more consuming. "It is through the constant frustration of desire that Late Capitalism can prompt ever higher levels of consumption." The fact that dieters end up being fatter after a while than they were before they began confirms the paradoxical logic that Schwartz uncovers.

"In such a society, sexism, racism, and class warfare would be unlikely."† Fat people are not hungry like imperialists, impatient like exploiters, intolerant or warlike. Schwartz concludes: "The

---

* Ibid., p. 328.
† Ibid., p. 330.

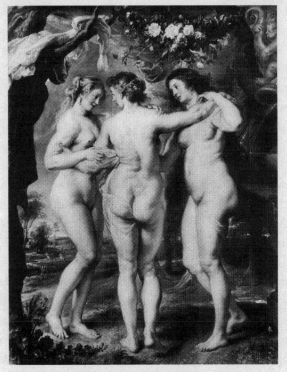

Three Graces *by Rubens*

most effective physiological method of making war impossible in future would be to organize a society for the universal diffusion of adipose."* If everyone were fat, the world would be fat and happy and peaceful, Schwartz thinks. Leanness is concomitant with meanness; fat brings peace and contentment to character.

* Ibid., p. 331.

Recommending that you EAT FAT seems irresponsible, on the face of it. In the face of the powerful forces

arrayed under the sign of health, it seems immoral to be seen to be encouraging people to do what they are already overdoing a lot. But you've already understood that my aim here is not to encourage obesity. This is a postmodern diet book, which starts on the other side of the realization that diets don't work. Even if your fat is unhealthy, which is far from being sure, trying to lose it will increase it in the long run, and may well do harm, in the meantime, to body and mind.

This discovery, which comes at the end of a century committed to dieting in the name of thin, has already begun to transform our consciousness. Or perhaps it is itself the sign of a new consciousness that will expand and develop in the next millennium as we progressively learn to EAT

FAT.

Suppose you credit the Body Image Task Force, a fat-acceptance group in California, and believe their claims are true: "Dieting has been shown to lead to anxiety, depression, lethargy, lowered self-esteem, decreased attention span, weakness, high blood pressure, hair loss, gall-bladder disease, gallstones, heart disease, ulcers, constipation, anemia, dry skin, skin rashes, dizziness, reduced sex drive, menstrual irregularities, amenorrhea, gout, infertility, kidney stones, numbness in the legs, weight gain, compulsive eating, anorexia nervosa, bulimia, reduced resistance to infection, lowered exercise tolerance, electrolyte imbalance, bone loss, osteoporosis and death."[*] If diets don't work and are bad for your health, what conclusions should we draw? The fat-acceptance movement draws the conclusion that we should give up trying to be thin and accept our fat. We should also demand tolerance from others. There is probably not much you can do if you're fat, they argue, so you might as well learn to live with it. And insist that others accept it. It is a whole other leap to the vision this book is trying to illuminate, a world in which fat once again has grown beautiful.

The fat-acceptance movement starts from the politically necessary assumption that society, which will never love fat, can at least learn to tolerate fatties. They themselves have personally experi-

---

[*] Body Image Task Force, P. O. Box 934, Santa Cruz, CA 95061.

enced the depth of sanctioned hatred directed against fat, which has become, for some, the last politically correct form of racism and discrimination. People, without hesitation, stigmatize the fat; they accuse them of sloth and self-indulgence, gluttony and loss of self-control. We are still allowed, in polite society, to hate fatties, because fat, it seems self-evident, is hateful.

But if we are all getting fatter, if diets don't work and do harm, what can we do, in the short term? We could start to love fat. Fat chance. But the diet industry has its own solutions in the works. If diets don't work, and amphetamines have been discredited, its answer is anorexiants, new kinds of drugs that make you thin. The word *anorexia* comes from the Greek and means without appetite or desire to eat. A whole generation of new drugs exploits recent discoveries about the mechanisms by which the body creates and accumulates fat.

The search for a silver bullet is on, one that will kill fat forever and allow all of us, regardless of our class or station, to be thin. In the meantime, there's a hot new development in diet "medicine," widespread in clinics sprung up around the country, where doctors prescribe a new generation of diet drugs that are serotonin stimulators. They are being peddled with vast unknown consequences for public health. While the diet merchants preach the unhealthiness of fat, they are selling diet drugs to an ever-growing segment of the population, and the possibilities in the future are enormous.

My position is this. Even if fat is unhealthy, which it is and it isn't, for the vast majority of people, it's probably healthier than the alternative. The alternative is dieting, compulsive exercise, hyper-vegetarianism, diet pills. My opinions start from the a priori premise that administering any powerful drugs to a large population over a long period of time is not good for public health.

It's true of course that many people take medicine to control their blood pressure and they take it for years. High blood pressure, like obesity, returns the minute you stop taking pills. But the comparison implies that fat, like high blood pressure, is itself a medical condition. Which it is and it isn't.

Some people are unhealthily fat.

Most fat people are perfectly healthy.

Suppose you believe like the hero of *The Confessions of Zeno,* a novel by Italo Svevo,* that health can be defined as mobility. He would say that you are healthy as long as you're moving. The minute fat, or anything else, impedes your mobility, limits your normal capacity freely, spontaneously to move, then, in my opinion, it is morbid. Morbid obesity is sometimes set at 100 pounds over your ideal or standard weight. But many people are perfectly healthy, many even happy, at that weight. Some people, by my definition, are morbidly fat, either because their fat is a physical impediment or because it directly contributes to some debilitating illnesses. The health of the morbid requires that they lose weight. Those people need to take heroic measures to reduce their body weight and cut fat.

But most people, who aren't morbidly obese, are fat for lots of reasons. Because they eat to deal with stress, or because their whole family is fat, or because they can't find time to exercise, or because the millennium approaches. Would it be a good thing if all these

*Italo Svevo, *The Confessions of Zeno* (New York: Random House, 1958).

people who are clinically obese, twenty pounds or more above their ideal weight, but otherwise perfectly healthy, were put on drugs that drastically changes metabolisms and alters mental states, in order to get the benefits of being thin? And, suppose these new drugs actually work. You can bet that most of the people taking them won't be doing it to improve their health. If drugs work, even top models will take them, not to mention all the other women (and men) who would kill to be thin—who would willingly pay substantial sums for their monthly diet fix. Over fifty million dieters—so many dieters, so little time.

The manufacturers of these new drugs need consequently to minimize the dangers of these drugs and to maximize the dangers of fat. They have an interest in persuading the medical profession, the public, and the FDA that any fat you bear increases your chances of dying young.

That's the conclusion that has been drawn from a recent, widely publicized study by Dr. JoAnn Manson, co-director of women's health at Brigham and Women's Hospital in Boston, an affiliate of Harvard Medical School. In her study,* published in the *New England Journal of Medicine*, Dr. Manson claims to have discovered, epidemiologically, a direct correlation between the body mass of middle-aged white women and their chances of early mortality. (Body mass is an expression of weight in relation to height.) Basically, the message is this: You can never be too thin. (Or too rich, it goes without saying.) Her conclusions are particularly depressing, at

*JoAnn E. Manson, et al., "Body Weight and Mortality Among Women," *New England Journal of Medicine* 333, no. 11 (September 14, 1995): 677–85.

a time when there has otherwise been a tendency to loosen "the iron maiden"—the constraining idea of "ideal weight" that has oppressed us all for so long. In recent years, a more liberal scale of "standard weight" has been taken up by doctors and actuaries, raising the bar—widening the waist of what is considered to be normal, what an average adult of a certain height is supposed to weigh. Along with that, doctors have also recently begun to take a somewhat more benign view of the place of fat in an overall interpretation of their patients' health. But Dr. Manson deplores this new permissiveness. "The increasingly permissive U.S. weight guidelines may therefore be unjustified and potentially harmful," she writes at the end of her report. She considers obese even the austere Mutual Insurance standards of ideal weight, last revised in 1957 and first proposed at the turn of the century. She told the *Atlanta Journal and Constitution*°: "Even average U.S. weights are 'overweight' when it comes to the risk of heart attack." In condemning the new permissiveness, Dr. Manson's wildly heralded conclusion coincides with the never-too-thin position of those in the beauty-health-fitness industry, who seek to banish fat by all and any means.

A cloud was cast over Dr. Manson's work when it was observed that, in addition to her research at Harvard, she works as a consultant to two companies manufacturing so-called obesity drugs. A footnote to her report indicates, for example, that she is "a scientific consultant" on "health effects of obesity for Interneuron Pharmaceutical in Lexington, Mass." Interneuron is a company seeking FDA approval of a new anorexiant drug, called dexfenfluramine. It

° *Atlanta Journal and Constitution,* February 8, 1995.

resembles the more familiar drug, fenfluramine, now in wide use in diet "clinics" (in conjunction with another drug, phentermine), but dex, as it's often called (inviting confusion with the amphetamine, Dexedrine), is more effective, with fewer side effects, and can be taken for much longer periods of time. Dr. Manson's connection to Interneuron is not uncommon. And unlike some, she makes no secret of her consulting, acknowledging in a footnote her ties to two companies that make diet pills. Companies regularly pay consultants who do studies and whose conclusions support the aims of the company. There's nothing illegal or unprofessional about that; it nevertheless permits suspicions to be aroused. There is a lot of pressure, unconscious or not, for statistical studies to be interpreted in ways that suit the prejudices or the commercial interests of the researcher.

Imagine you were the owner of a hot pharmaceutical firm that had the right to produce and was now seeking to market a powerful obesity drug. Suppose you watched nervously as people, growing fatter, became more tolerant of fat, while you're waiting years for FDA approval. Aren't you hoping in your heart of hearts that science will prove what you already profoundly believe, every pound of fat lost enhances your shot at longevity? Wouldn't it be in your company's interest to be able to cite scientific evidence that every pound gained increases your mortal risk? As the owner and operator of such a drug firm, wouldn't you be pleased to learn this good news from a person you were consulting, were paying to be "a scientific consultant," as Interneuron does with Dr. Manson? The thrilling results of her Harvard statistics are clear: More fat, more risk. Period.

You might come home to your wife, who is also your partner in the firm, and say, Hey! Honey, look at this. You know that consultant we paid for. She's just published a paper in a respected scientific-medical journal demonstrating that with every pound of fat you lose you lower your chance of dying young. Would that be a good day or not? Damn, if all along doctors haven't been right to scold! No one has the right to be complacent about plump or happy with a few extra pounds. That sort of fat acceptance belonged to a brief moment of permissiveness in the early nineties. New science tells us that the old strictness must return, with a vengeance. Science and authority come together to serve each other, to make money and murder fat.

Not all experts, however, agree with Dr. Manson. A recent study by Dr. David Heymsfield suggests that being slightly over-weight after seventy poses no additional dangers; whereas, conversely, being thinner than normal entails a greater risk.° Risk of what? A statistical risk of dying early. That is what the researchers measure. The study by Dr. Heymsfield of St. Luke's-Roosevelt Hospital in New York used statistical methods similar to those employed by Dr. Manson of Harvard, but their conclusions lend themselves to very different interpretations.

But suppose you tried to reconcile the seemingly contradictory conclusions of these two extensive studies, 7,000 men and women in one case, 200,000 nurses in the other. Taken together they seem to say, If you're fat, you may not live to seventy, but if you do, you'll live even longer, being fat, than if you were thin. So the rule of

° *New York Times,* October 18, 1995.

hygiene would seem to be: Be extremely thin when it's hard to lose weight, but after sixty-five, when the body loses weight anyway from muscle and bone—then, when it's easier to be thin, be fat. If you want to live long, assuming that's your goal, be thin when it's easy to be fat, and fat when it's easy to be thin.

The conclusions drawn by Dr. Heymsfield's study are compatible, the *New York Times* reports, with earlier studies suggesting that the "weight associated with the lowest mortality risk also increased gradually with age." That means, the weight of the people who live longest goes up, particularly among the elderly. But that view of things is also questioned in the *Times,* by another doctor, Bray, who thinks that it may be a statistical illusion. Since a lot of really fat people have already died by the age of seventy, the ones left who are fat are just lucky. They probably shouldn't have survived for so long. If you get to be seventy and are still fat, then you've beaten longer odds than you think. But now that you've gotten there, fat, you'll probably live longer than if you were thin.

What are the odds that you will die earlier than you might if you weighed twenty or thirty pounds less than what you currently weigh? According to Dr. Manson's own study, there is only an insignificantly greater risk of a middle-aged woman dying young who weighs twenty to thirty pounds above her ideal weight. Most overweight middle-aged women don't die young. They die when they are old.

But suppose you decide to improve your risks, and lose twenty to thirty pounds. Suppose you go on a rigorous diet, lose weight, keep it off, get happy and live longer. How likely is it that will happen? If you get serious and decide to submit yourself to a rigorous diet, you may be doing yourself a lot more harm than if you had incurred the greater risk of staying fat and dying young. You really ought to assume that if you start, you'll give it up, much before anything like thirty pounds disappears. Even if you briefly accomplish your goal, even if you lose thirty pounds, you run enormous risks of being a whole lot fatter three or four years down the road. In the meantime you've brutalized your body and agonized under the pain of diets and exercise, guilt, disappointment, anxiety, anger. You are probably eating badly—fetishistically and without any taste. You've made yourself unhappy and disagreeable and unpleasured and you are bound in the end to get fatter. Your dieting could be the prelude to serious eating disorders—to eating perversions like anorexia and bulimia, where food is so much an issue for the dieter, becomes so highly symbolic, that it is negatively eroticized: it comes to be what you love to hate. Food, for example, for many adolescent girls is their parents. Dieting may provoke a perversion in your attitude toward eating and poisons life. The question remains: Should a middle-aged woman endanger her health and happiness by dieting, in order to lose enough weight to diminish her already small risk of dying early?

Dr. Manson's and Dr. Heymsfield's studies are based on what is called the observational method. A researcher studies a coherent group of people, called a cohort, over a long period of time. The aim of this statistical study is to seek correlations between risk factors, like being fat and cigarette smoking, and whatever health problems develop in the group. Epidemiological studies like these rely heavily on subjects in the group reporting information themselves, in questionnaires they send back to the researcher. Naturally, this sort of information is not always reliable, although conscientious scientists take precautions against its defects. Most people, for example, lie about their weight by about six pounds, as a general rule. And many studies correct for that. It goes without saying that in our society, people always lie in the direction of seeming to be thinner than they are. Even science takes it for granted that in our society no one would ever lie about being thin and exaggerate their weight, unless they were anorexic. It's funny to think that a century ago, when men and women dreamt of abundant décolletages, when corpulent men were admired and desired, scientists might have started with precisely the opposite self-evident assumption. People back then would have exaggerated their weight upward. No one at the turn of the century would have desired to be thin.

In 1976, the Nurses Health Study pool was established, when 121,700 female registered nurses thirty to fifty-five years of age, who lived in eleven states mostly in the East, responded to questionnaires requesting information about their medical history and health behavior. Dr. Manson indicates in her notes that 98 percent of that population was white. It is, of course, widely recognized that African- and Hispanic-American women are as a whole much fatter than white women, and thus generally healthier at higher weights. But Dr. Manson in stating her conclusions doesn't emphasize the race factors in her study.

In this survey, there were 115,195 mostly white middle-class, middle-aged U.S. women, between thirty and fifty-five, free of known cardiovascular disease and cancer in 1976 (when the study began). Obviously, some of this disease was present though unknown to the nurses at the time the study began. During the sixteen-year span, 4,726 women died, 18 percent from heart disease, 54 percent from cancer, and the rest from other causes. After analyzing the data, Dr. Manson concluded that of those who didn't smoke or have any major diseases (cardiovascular diseases or cancer), there was a statistical correlation between early mortality and fat. The thinner you were the less likely you were to die young.

You have to notice first of all that among all those women, only 4 percent died. 96 percent of the women—fat or thin—didn't die. So this study measures the relative risks of these women dying during sixteen years of their middle age when the absolute risk is low anyway. Some of them could be as old as fifty-five plus sixteen years, or seventy-one, when they died; yet their death counts in determining the general mortality of the pool—the chance of their dying during middle age—making the risks seem even greater than they are. For most, dying young after seventy is not seen as a particularly great risk.

Besides, in drawing conclusions from the pool, Manson considered non-smokers apart. She writes: "When women who had never smoked were examined separately, no increase in risk was observed among the leaner women, and a more direct relation between weight and mortality emerged." In other words, once you eliminate from the group of thin women those who smoke, and those who harbor heart disease, cancer or other major illnesses, the remainder are less likely to die soon. But of course a lot of women smoke in order to be thin. In fact, Dr. Manson found that current smokers constituted 43.8 percent of the thinnest group of women, almost half of them, while only 23.3 percent of the heaviest nurses smoked. In other words, almost half the women who were "ideally" thin, according to Manson's conclusions, were thin and smoked, which of course is much worse for your health than being fat. And it was the fattest women who were the least likely to smoke, which is good for your health. But of course, thin and smoking is a lot riskier than fat and smoke free. If, statistically, you want to die young, smoke.

Perhaps the fattest people in general are healthier than the thinnest people, in general, since the latter are much more likely to smoke. But Dr. Manson didn't ask the question. Her interest focused on the group of nurses who never smoked and whose weight never fluctuated more than twenty pounds after the age of twenty. She triumphantly concludes that those genetically thin, non-smoking women, who have never had to diet, had less chance of dying young than any of the others. Abstracting from a group with these good genes and these good habits, Manson concludes that you can never be too thin.

You can understand why some doctors worried, at the time of the publication, that the effect of Manson's study would be to encourage women, in particular, in their pursuit of thinness at any cost. Her conclusion, based on this select group of women, risks reinforcing the wishful belief that there's some advantage in living like models, on coffee and Marlboros. Alcohol consumption was also more common among the thinner women, which suggests that one way to be thin is to become an alcoholic. Drunks don't eat much.

One of Dr. Manson's surprising discoveries was that while hypertension, diabetes, and elevated serum cholesterol were two to six times more prevalent in the heaviest categories, there was very little difference among the women of all sizes in the amount of fat they actually ate. In other words, fat women got fat eating no more fat than many thin women eat. Their bodies made more fat with the same food.

In the view of some of the epidemiologists who met recently with journalists in Boston, the Manson study illustrates the tendency among scientists to overstate their findings, confusing the public. "By one day saying one thing, the next another, we are in collusion with the confusion," said Dr. Charles H. Hennekens, a professor of epidemiology at Harvard University's School of Public Health, noted for a study showing aspirin's benefit in reducing the risk of heart disease. "Epidemiology is a crude and inexact science. . . . We tend to overstate findings, either because we want attention or more grant money."[*] Journalists naturally tingle at the titillating conclusions that scientists hype—focusing their articles on whatever in the study can be taken to be hot and new. The public gets what it deserves and expects, dreams of a quick fix for their anxiety over fat and promises of magical solutions to the puzzle of losing weight. Most newspaper reports of Manson's study transmitted its conclusions with emphasis on the 5'5", 119-pound level at which the death risk was lowest. Even though, for example, black women of the same height and weight don't face at all the same risks as white women. Neither, for that matter, do smokers, or heavy drinkers, or yo-yo dieters.

The pitfalls of epidemiological research are many. In the case of the nurses, it is not only that they might be inclined to lie, like many women, about their weight. But they are also a cohort who

[*] *New York Times*, October 11, 1995.

know, or think they know, what the researcher is looking to find. It's not too surprising if their report on themselves, white middle-aged, middle-class nurses, reflects the general attitudes toward health you might expect in a group of people like that at this period in America. This particular period in fact corresponds to the moment that Roberta Seid, the great historian of dieting, describes in the section of her book, "From Myth to Obsession: 1970–1980." She writes, "A fundamental difference between the seventies and the previous two decades was the emergence of health-consciousness as an ethical principle. . . . We came to believe that the typical American diet—high in fat, salt, meat, and refined sugar—was not only fattening but also unhealthy in and of itself.* Eating fat was not only likely to lead to being fat, but fat was a kind of moral poison.

Endocrinologist Dr. Dianne Budd of Women's Health Access at the University of California San Francisco, was one of those who expressed concern that the Harvard study might lure women into radical diets or fasting in order to achieve the lowest risk condition, the body mass index corresponding to 5'5", 119 pounds. Dr. Budd knows that obtaining and maintaining a weight 15 percent beneath the average weight of most women entails fasting and diets so radical as to do more harm to your health and happiness than would settling for the fat you've got. Dr. Budd argues that the Harvard study focused on "a magical subset of women" who were genetically programmed to be thin—congenitally healthy, stable, and thin. "They're about 10 percent of the population," says Budd. "And

* Seid, p. 165.

none of those are my patients!"* Yet, on National Public Radio's "All Things Considered,"† JoAnn Manson summed up her study in these words: "Based on these findings, about one-quarter of all deaths in women are attributable to overweight, making obesity second only to cigarette smoking as a preventable cause of premature death" Dr. Manson has taken another step in the medicalization of fat, on the way to its politicization. Fat has been made murderous, hardly less venomous than nicotine, another deadly poison, which kills large rats in minute doses. And like cigarette smoking, obesity, says Dr. Manson, as if it were a matter of fact— as if it goes without saying—is preventable. It might be inferred from these conclusions that the government ought to intervene to combat the public health dangers of fat, first by declaring it a drug requiring regulation, then by approving new drugs to reduce the dangers of obesity, while encouraging anorexiant manufacturers. From here it's just a step to the view of Kelly D. Brownell, the often quoted Yale professor of psychology and nutrition, who wants taxes imposed on fatty foods.

But, after all, what does preventable mean—exactly? For the people, say, at Interneuron who financed Dr. Manson's study, "preventable" does not merely mean that you can cut fat by diets and exercise, which don't work. Fat will be preventable, for many or most people, thanks to a pill.

Interneuron is a controversial company founded in 1988 by Richard and Judith Wurtman, two researchers at MIT, who own the

---

* *San Francisco Examiner,* October 8, 1995.

† National Public Radio, "All Things Considered," September 13, 1995.

U.S. patent to commercialize dexfenfluramine, a diet drug manufactured by the French pharmaceutical firm Servier Amérique. Dex, as it's known on Wall Street, made Interneuron a sexy company, when it went public in 1990, turning the Wurtmans into paper millionaires, according to the *Wall Street Journal.*[*] Just last November a committee at the FDA recommended that dexfenfluramine be approved for distribution in the United States. By now it has begun to be sold in prescription under the brand name Redux.

In the late 1960s Americans were consuming vast amounts of amphetamine, forms of speed, which doctors often prescribed without even examining their patients.[†] By the end of the seventies the euphoria wore off. Not only did people gain weight back the instant they stopped popping pills, a lot of people couldn't stop the pop. Many became addicted, some were suicidal, few benefited over the long term from doing daily doses of speed. Eventually, doctors who continued to prescribe amphetamines came to be viewed as slightly sleazy, since the pill they promoted was so liable to abuse. People hooked on speed are perfectly thin, but as is usually the case, being perfectly thin means paying a terrible price. Bodies hooked on diets of speed eventually succumb to the intense acceleration of their metabolism by breaking down in first subtle, then devastating ways. And coming down from speed is always a bummer. So the medical profession in general, and the FDA in particular, has been until now resisting applications for approval of a new generation of drugs. They have taken the position that obesity

[*] *Wall Street Journal,* July 20, 1994.
[†] Seid, p. 138.

is a matter of behavior, of will and self-control, that drugs are only temporarily useful. Since you cannot treat a moral problem with short-term drugs, the only answer the FDA provides has been the oldest nostrum in the book: diet and exercise.

The person perhaps most responsible for this renewed interest on the part of doctors in treating obesity with drugs is Dr. Michael Weintraub, a clinical pharmacologist, at the University of Rochester Medical School. He questioned the current, orthodox medical fashion disapproving the use of drugs, and showed the effectiveness of a program including diet, exercise, and two appetite-reducing chemical substances. Dr. Weintraub in his study administered a new class of anorexiants to eighty-one people, who, in his professional opinion, needed to lose weight in order to reduce hypertension, high cholesterol, diabetes, or some other medical condition.

In his paper, Dr. Weintraub addresses the nature of the skepticism, widespread throughout the medical profession, concerning the use of anorexiants. In a passage that sounds surprisingly like an appeal for fat acceptance, he denounces his medical colleagues and indicts society for the moral stigma it attaches to obesity. His diagnosis of the general "lack of understanding" of obesity implies a revolution in medical attitudes. Here is what Dr. Weintraub, a doctor and teacher of doctors, writes:

> Both the medical profession and society look with disfavor on obese people and obesity in general. For example, students at a well-known university preferred a number of less savory people to obese individuals as potential partners. Obese people are treated negatively in cartoons and in literature. Many

believe that obese people need only to "close their mouths" and be more motivated to lose weight. Thus use of medications to correct a characterological defect is, in the opinion of physicians and the public, deemed inappropriate.*

Many fat-acceptance advocates have been documenting for years the mistreatment suffered by the obese at the hands of the medical profession. It's surprising to hear a teacher of doctors confirming the analysis of those who say that the profession has been ferociously demonizing fat for a century—for reasons that are not fully medical. In fact, Dr. Weintraub is confirming the whole powerful feminist argument that recommendations to lose weight coming from doctors are often unscientific, frequently moralizing, cruelly patronizing, a sanctioned form of harassment. Doctors themselves are prejudiced by the ideal of body weight we have come to construct in this century. For all too many doctors, fat is a matter of character and you are a better person, a more responsible adult, the more nearly you conform to the ideal—to their idea of ideal weight.

Dr. Weintraub implies that too many doctors share with adolescents the most extreme forms of fatphobia. Fat for both may be more unsavory (although it tastes good) than crime or moral decay. Dr. Weintraub castigates his medical colleagues for sharing in the caricature of fat, in the negative treatment it receives at the

---

* Michael Weintraub, M.D., "Introduction. Long-term Weight Control: The National Heart, Lung, and Blood Institute Funded Multimodal Intervention Study." *Clinical Pharmacological Therapy* 51, no. 5 (May 1992): 582.

hands of popular culture, "in cartoons and in literature," he writes.° It's true you sometimes see cartoons where the fat are ridiculous or read fiction where they are preposterous. But I wonder what literature the doctor reads, which cartoons he means. Fat Albert, after all, is adorable. Mr. Pickwick is memorable.

Dr. Weintraub makes contemptuous fun of his medical colleagues, who so stigmatize fat with their moral disapproval that they don't even consider it a medical problem at all. For them it's a matter of self-control—the problem of patients who can't "close their mouths." It's like a doctor telling patients who come for birth control that all they really need to do is keep their legs together. For these doctors, being fat is like being pregnant; it's a moral choice, not a medical problem.

Having denounced medicine's "pejorative view" of obesity, after confirming what we have long suspected, Dr. Weintraub draws a surprising, disappointing conclusion. You might expect that since he has the same diagnosis as fat acceptance, he would embrace its remedies. You might think that if doctors gave up their caricatures of fat people, if they stopped thinking fat was a matter of character—if they started looking at reality instead of swallowing caricatures and fictions about fat—you might think it would lead to some fat acceptance. Instead, he draws from the same premise a radically different therapeutic conclusion. It allows him to conclude that, because of their unscientific prejudices, doctors have been insufficiently willing to prescribe drugs for obesity. For, according to Dr. Weintraub, their prejudice against fat also takes the form of

° Ibid.

a bias directed against anorexiants. If doctors didn't hate fat, didn't make it a moral issue, they would recognize that diets don't work, and they would look for better drugs to give their patients. Dr. Weintraub ends up prescribing pills.

He ends up promoting drugs for those who have a distinct, compelling medical reason for losing weight. He writes, "The benefits of losing some weight and maintaining that loss are potentially very great. A small weight loss may suffice in helping to control elevated blood pressure, blood sugar (in adult-onset diabetes), and cholesterol."[*]

Diets don't work, pills do. Recognizing that, Dr. Weintraub medicalizes weight loss. He takes it out of the moral sphere, where recommendations to diet and exercise are not medicine but pastoral guidance. He focuses on medical means for achieving a specific weight loss, in the interest of what he calls very great benefits to people with certain conditions. He is quite clear about his justification for administering drugs to a group of people over a long period of time, and warns against the dangers of their misuse: "Attempting to induce greater changes in body weight for cosmetic or purported health benefits may be counterproductive because failure will be inevitable, the regain of lost weight will be highly likely, and the potential for a 'roller coaster' or 'yo-yo' situation will be created." Naturally, Dr. Weintraub distinguishes himself from pill-meisters, from all those doctors in Hollywood and Palm Beach who can't say no to their wealthy clients, for whom a pill to be thin is a cosmetic dream come true. But you notice he's also careful to

[*] Ibid., p. 644.

stay away from the raging debate about the health benefits of thin. He avoids the questions raised by Dr. Manson's claims concerning the purported health benefits, the lowered risk of mortality, from being thin. Dr. Weintraub's medical intervention has modest aims. To help the people with chronic conditions and serious diseases who need to lose pounds.

Dr. Weintraub's experimental study was a modest but unmistakable success. Most people lost weight and maintained the loss as long as they kept taking the pills. The majority of subjects rapidly gained weight when they stopped taking their medicine, even those who continued to exercise and continued to follow their controlled diet. The participants in the study did not reach their ideal weight. Most reduced their body weight by an average of 10–15 percent during the period they took their medicine.

Roughly 15 percent of the group dropped out of the program because of the drugs' adverse side effects. They included dry mouth, but most important, sleep disturbances. Participants suffered from difficulty falling asleep, excessive sleepiness, disturbed sleep, and vivid dreams. Some mentioned nervousness and "tension"; a few experienced cardiovascular symptoms like increased blood pressure, palpitations, or irregular heart rhythm, but these were rare. Many participants mentioned adverse symptoms, but most found them tolerable over the period of several years. When the drugs were stopped suddenly and then resumed, the adverse effects seemed to be worse.

Dr. Weintraub sums up one of the lessons he learned from this study: "We must teach ourselves and our patients to measure success by prevention of weight gain and maintenance of a significant but perhaps more modest weight loss than we or they would find 'desirable.' "[*]

Yet, despite the modesty of Dr. Weintraub's ambitions and the slimness of his results, his work has been enormously influential. According to the *Wall Street Journal,* the study "set off a tidal wave when it was published in the May 1992 issue of the journal *Clinical Pharmacology and Therapeutics.* Thousands of doctors besieged Dr. Weintraub for copies."[†] The drugs have now been administered to tens of thousands of people, and the drug companies have added extra shifts to produce vast quantities of drugs that had been languishing on shelves for years. Suddenly, despite Dr. Weintraub's modesty, drugs again were hot.

In my local newspaper today there is an ad for a "Medical Weight Loss Center" with a headline that says: "Diets Don't Work." It's the same premise as Dr. Weintraub's. Dr. Weintraub writes: "We proposed a long-term study because we viewed obesity as a chronic condition that should be treated over a substantial period of time."[‡] The ad seems to echo that conclusion—rather more forcefully, and with a whole other implication: "Being chronically overweight is a disease. Weight control is not a problem of sheer will power—it's a disease that begins in a part of the brain that controls hunger. Like other diseases, it is a medical problem with a medical solution," says the advertisement. Nothing in the ad limits the "patient" pool to those who have medical problems, like high blood pressure or dia-

[*] Ibid.
[†] July 20, 1994.
[‡] Ibid.

betes, which reducing fat might alleviate. Obesity itself has become
a disease that these doctors promise to remedy. The ad screams,
"Lose Weight Now and Keep It Off Long Term." Nowhere do they
say that if you stop taking these pills after a few months, as you must,
you'll probably regain your weight and then some.

Dr. Weintraub warned against using these drugs for cosmetic
purposes. No such warnings are given by the diet center advertisement. To qualify for the program you have only to be between eighteen and sixty, pass a physical, and be 20 percent over your ideal
weight. That restriction may well be intended to discourage those
whose interests in losing weight are mainly cosmetic or obsessive,
like those of anorexics, who always think they need to lose a few
more pounds. But on the right side of the ad is a chart of "Ideal
Body Weight" that reproduces one of the most restrictive versions
of the grid defining "ideal weight." This iron maiden, for example,
puts the ideal weight of a woman 5′ 5″ at 125 pounds, and of a man
5′ 9″ at 155. To me that's skinny. The ad never promises that you will
be able to achieve that ideal weight, but it reports a "93 percent success rate" among patients taking drugs.

I called up the weight center and asked them which drugs they
were using. They were the same as those prescribed by Dr. Weintraub. Nothing suggests that these drugs are being administered to
achieve the narrow aims that Dr. Weintraub describes. On the contrary, it's clear that a lot of money is being made feeding pills to
people who hate their fat.

Dr. Weintraub's views are echoed by Dr. Douglas Green of the
FDA, who is quoted in the *Wall Street Journal* saying: "Obesity
used to be viewed as a lack of willpower in a patient. It was not

viewed as a medical problem. Today I think it is."* Douglas Green is an endocrinologist at the University of Michigan who heads an FDA committee of outside experts that studies new obesity drugs. About them, he said, "There are many that are under development, and our hope is that we would be able to get such agents to add to our armamentarium." The weaponry of obesity drugs will soon be even more widely deployed in a war against fat—that most preventable cause of premature death.

In 1992 Dr. Weintraub became the director of the FDA's office of over-the-counter drug evaluation. It may be no coincidence that since then the FDA has become increasingly receptive to the arguments of companies eager to market diet drugs.

The drugs Dr. Weintraub chose for his study were two. One was an appetite suppressant that had been well known to this clinical pharmacologist. It is an earlier, cruder appetite suppressant, manufactured by Fisons PLC, called Ionamin. The other was a drug manufactured by the A. H. Robins Company, Pondimin, which had the effect of raising levels of serotonin, a substance in the brain that seems particularly devoted to regulating mood. These drugs have become widely known by their chemical names, phentermine and fenfluramine. The companies that make them had virtually stopped marketing them; now their stocks are booming.

Dr. Weintraub believes that if "obesity is a chronic condition, shouldn't it need chronic treatment. Nobody would ever say a blood-pressure drug didn't work if a patient's blood pressure went

---

* *Wall Street Journal,* July 20, 1994.

back up when he stopped taking it."[*] Weintraub's conception is also supported by Manson's study. If obesity is a chronic condition, the second highest cause of premature death, then doesn't it need a medical solution in the form of a drug that works long term? The longer you stay thin the more you lower your risk of dying early. So why not take a drug that makes you thin to make your death less premature?

The possibility that a drug raising serotonin levels might cut appetite, reduce craving, is one that has been recognized relatively recently. These drugs operate on a biological principle different from, say, amphetamines, that speed up the body's metabolism, as well as the mind. The new drugs work to calm the stressed mind of overeaters, which sends urgent signals to eat in the form of cravings whenever the system wants a little boost in well-being or pleasure. The theory behind these drugs has come to see food itself as a drug, as a mild narcotic or stimulant, a mood enhancer or antidepressant, a mild hallucinogen or narcotic. The body uses food to alter its state of mind, to re-establish chemical imbalances that one experiences as sudden urges or persistent cravings to eat.

The development of this whole line of drugs starts from scientific premises quite different from those that direct the search for a fat gene. That other, more fundamental research is looking for a hormone that will tell the body to stop making fat. But at the origin of the attempt to develop these new Prozac-like drugs is an interest in the fact that men and women, although to different degrees, have uncontrollable, insatiable cravings. What is a craving?

[*] Weintraub, p. 582.

Food and mood are linked. Eat a bagel and relax, says Judith Wurtman wearing her MIT nutritionist hat. Eat any carbohydrates, from simple sugars to grains and pastas, and your brain produces serotonin. Describing a path first fully traced by her husband and partner, Dr. Richard Wurtman, she elucidates the conversion from bagel to bliss. First, the body converts the bagel's starch to sugar. The sugar prompts the pancreas to produce insulin; insulin raises brain levels of an amino acid, tryptophan, which in turn triggers serotonin, a neurotransmitter, which decreases pain and helps induce calm and drowsiness—which makes you feel "more emotionally comfortable." Faced with stress, chewing a bagel at the right moment will give your body a natural tranquilizer that reduces its craving for carbohydrates. Some fat people need a drug to stop the craving brought on by insufficient serotonin, as the body seeks a way to calm its tension and ease the pain.

The Wurtman theory is that you eat fat to feel good. In other words, food is the ultimate drug, the high to which we are all addicted. Some of us can't get enough of the good feeling, and so we overeat. In order to stop doing food, goes the theory, take drugs. The minute food is understood to be a drug, another drug will be found to counter its effects.

Protein helps produce two other neurotransmitters—dopamine and norepinephrine—which tend to stimulate alertness, improve concentration, and accelerate rates of reaction. Fat, conversely, slows the production of dopamine and norepinephrine, so chicken soup is soporific. But while fat doesn't seem to have any effect on the production of serotonin, it does work to stimulate the production of endorphins in the brain, natural substances with pain-killing properties whose chemical action resembles that of morphine. Dr. Adam Drewnowski of the University of Michigan thinks that what both men and women want is pleasure: "Fat makes you feel good." He says that cravings in people who eat normal diets are not nutritional, but that does not mean such needs are all bad: studies show that pleasure releases endorphins, strengthening the immune system.*

What conclusion could one draw from this? Suppose you were suffering from PMS. Just before your period, your endorphin level has dropped after hitting a high during ovulation. You feel the usual irritated boredom, the slight depression and fatigue that make you doubt yourself and your powers. The answer, as Debra Waterhouse has argued in her book *Why Women Love Chocolate,* is three Hershey kisses.† Eaten in the afternoon when your body hits chemical bottom, the sugar and the fat in the chocolate, plus other substances, combine to raise the levels of the chemicals that make you feel good. The sugar prompts the production of serotonin, and the fat releases endorphins producing a feeling of calm. Chocolate contains caffeine and phenylethylamine, or PEA, thought to stimulate the release of endorphins in the brain, which ease the pain. Suddenly, life once more has meaning. You don't need a lot of Hershey kisses to get the high. As with most drugs, you can maintain at low levels if you pay attention to the high and cultivate it. The trouble is that most of us want more and more. Three kisses can be the overture to an operatic orgy of bingeing on chocolate, leaving you no

* *The Commercial Appeal,* March 16, 1995.

† Debra Waterhouse, *Why Women Love Chocolate: Eat What You Crave to Look and Feel Great* (New York: Hyperion, 1995).

better off than before, worse in fact, engulfed by guilt and self-loathing.

Waterhouse recognizes that men generally have a different relation to chocolate. Men don't usually need it the way women do; they need other things to make them feel good. Judith Wurtman thinks that men, ruled by testosterone, require more protein to build and synthesize muscle, which would explain their cravings for meat, hot dogs, and eggs.* I think it's not the protein so much as the fat in meat men love. Not fat and sugar, but fat and salt is what I mostly crave.

The Wurtman theory of dieting sees serotonin production as the key to weight loss. Raising the serotonin level increases our feelings of well-being and consequently damps our cravings for food. Dr. Weintraub's treatment uses a long-known serotonin enhancer, the compound fenfluramine. The Wurtmans' drug, dexfenfluramine, is only half the molecule, but the business half—the part that increases serotonin without the occasional side effects: the dry mouth, dizziness, diarrhea, unsteadiness and memory problems associated with the older Weintraub formula, the one currently being prescribed. What's more, dex can be taken for much longer periods of time, without apparent ill effects, to judge by reports from Europe, where it has been legally available for some time. What's more, there's no disputing that it works for lots of people as long as they keep on taking it. It cuts appetite and cuts craving. People frequently lose 12 percent to 18 percent of their body weight on a regime of dexfenfluramine.

* Judith Wurtman, quoted in the *New York Times*, March 16, 1995.

One troubling question arises. How long can you take this drug, and what are its long-term effects? Warnings about the long-term dangers of dex have not been long in coming. Two studies by researchers at Johns Hopkins Hospital in Baltimore have demonstrated, in rats and squirrel monkeys, that administering doses of the drug large enough to suppress appetite produces toxic changes in the brain, specifically in brain serotonin neurons. Continued taking of oral dex kills the cells that produce serotonin in these laboratory animals—not only in rats, which metabolize the drug like humans, but in monkeys, which are primates like us.

A recent study, "Dexfenfluramine and Serotonin Neurotoxicity: Further Preclinical Evidence that Clinical Caution Is Indicated," concludes with this warning:

> Taken together, these findings indicate that concern over possible dexfenfluramine neurotoxicity in humans is warranted, and that physicians and patients alike need to be aware of dexfenfluramine's toxic potential toward brain serotonin neurons.[*]

The Endrocronolic and Metabolic Committee of the FDA met on November 16 and 17, 1995, in order to vote on whether they would recommend approving the licensing of dexfenfluramine. The vote was six to five in favor of approval. The close vote reflects the uneasiness of many in the scientific community about possible side effects attributed to dex. At the November meeting, the FDA committee listened to expert witnesses who testified on both sides

---

[*] *Journal of Pharmacology and Experimental Therapeutics* 269, no. 2 (1994): 792.

of the question of safety. One witness from the Clinical Trials Branch of the National Diabetes Center, Dr. Ron Innerfields, concluded his testimony saying,

> Dexfenfluramine causes pulmonary hypertension, which is both lethal and debilitating. Its long-term benefits have yet to be established. It is both unsafe and ineffective. It should simply not be approved.[*]

Dr. Innerfields concluded his report to the committee with a ringing assertion of the motto, to which all doctors are supposed to ascribe, *Premium no nocari.* (First of all, do no harm.)

The sponsor of dexfenfluramine, Interneuron Pharmaceuticals Incorporated, presented new testimony to the committee, claiming to demonstrate that dex was effective and posed little risk. The main spokesperson for Interneuron was Dr. Glen Cooper who began by citing the epidemic of obesity that was threatening public health in America. At one point he says, "Approximately 300,000 excess deaths per year are attributable to obesity, making obesity the second leading cause of preventable death, behind cigarette smoking. We're in the midst of a bona fide public health epidemic in this country."[†] He refers the committee members to the study that had already been presented to them by Dr. JoAnn E. Manson from Boston. What is more, "Dr. Manson is here today to answer questions," he adds.[‡]

---

[*] *Minutes of the Endrocronolic and Metabolic Committee of the FDA,* p. 52.

[†] Ibid., p. 69.

[‡] Ibid.

Dr. Cooper dismisses as statistically insignificant the small number of cases when people taking dexfenfluramine died from a sudden excess of pulmonary hypertension. He presents evidence that no neurological or psychological alteration in humans taking dex has been observed. Finally, he turns to counter the most powerful argument against approving the drug, that long-term use in animals at high doses produces irrefutable evidence on autopsy of toxic changes in the brain neurons that produce serotonin, causing "significant and in some cases prolonged reduction in brain serotonin content," as even the sponsor Interneuron agrees.* Against this clearly demonstrable fact in animals, Dr. Cooper musters a variety of arguments. The "axon tangles" or brain cell twisting the committee saw resulted not from dex but from taking Ecstacy. The brain changes that occur are undeniable, but are not necessarily toxic. And most telling in his arsenal is the argument over doses. Dr. Cooper, speaking for Interneuron, argued that prolonged use of dexfenfluramine is safe in humans at recommended doses much lower in relation to body weight than the high doses administered to animals, whose brains showed signs of poisoning. "There is a large margin of safety between clinically recommended doses and the doses that produce prolonged serotonin depletion in animals," he asserts.† At one point a note of something like paranoia creeps into the tone of Dr. Cooper, at the moment he is talking about the researchers who have found evidence of neurotoxicity in animals, rats and squirrel monkeys, receiving their high doses of dex. Dr. Cooper asks, "Why

* Ibid., pp. 82–83.
† Ibid., p. 86.

do they use doses that large?" His answer is slightly bizarre, "Because they do not see the long-term changes they want to see with lower doses, or, more importantly, with continuous administration of the drug."* He is accusing the researchers of having a pre-existing disposition to want to discredit dexfenfluramine. For what reason? Why would these big, bad researchers, academic scientists with impeccable, distinguished reputations, like Dr. Louis Seiden of the University of Chicago or Dr. George Ricaurte at Johns Hopkins, falsify their results by administering inappropriately high doses to their animals? What interest could they have in wanting to see long-term changes, when they didn't show up at first at lower doses? It is hard to imagine that these researchers had any motive in their work other than wanting to protect the public health against the long-term effects of administering a powerful drug over a long period of time to potentially enormous numbers of people here and around the world. They must certainly have weighed the dangers inherent in making widely available an effective pill for dieting, that over time might kill brain cells. Surely they thought about the passionate enthusiasm with which people will take up these pills, if they are deemed to be safe by the FDA. Think of the money that can be made from the misuse of a drug that pretty much ensures a limited but significant weight loss, with few side effects, and with no need to drastically restrict diet or increase activity. What venal or self-deluded or unprofessional motive is being implicitly attributed to these researchers by Dr. Cooper? Why would they risk their reputations to ensure the existence of evidence proving what they wanted

* Ibid., p. 85.

in advance to find: that dex is bad for your brain? By contrast, of course, Interneuron has no interest at all in seeing scientific results that confirm the conclusions they ardently wish for.

I asked George Ricaurte at Johns Hopkins University, one of the lead researchers in two of the animal studies of dex, what motive he had for finding "Further Preclinical Evidence That Clinical Caution Is Indicated," as one of the articles is subtitled.* He admitted to being puzzled by my question. He thought the sponsor, Interneuron, had made the FDA committee dizzy under an avalanche of data and its subtle interpretations. The simple fact remains, said Dr. Ricaurte, that in every animal species to which dexfenfluramine has been administered in doses high enough to produce weight loss, neurotoxicity can be observed on autopsy. Anorectic doses are neurotoxic in all the animals studied. Until autopsies are performed on humans who have taken dex for a long time, what perfect assurance can the FDA give that the dex effect won't be the same on human brains? Why take chances on a massive scale with human neurons, until proof of dex's safety can be unambiguously established? The answer, my friends, is the so-called epidemic of obesity, which takes over 300,000 lives a year, the second most common cause of premature death after smoking. If dexfenfluramine in high doses is poison, fat in even modest amounts is a killer. The FDA committee voted six to five to recommend approval. Several members changed their earlier vote. A final decision by the agency is not expected before fall, 1996.[†] There's little doubt the committee members were moved by

---

* *Journal of Pharmocology and Experimental Therapeutics* 269, no. 2 (1994): 792.

[†] Approval came earlier than expected, in May 1996.

a sense of duty to do something to halt the explosion of fat that has occurred in this country. They might also have been aware of the recent criticism directed at the FDA for being too slow, too reluctant to make available to an avid public some of the newest and most cunning products of a booming pharmaceutical industry. Once that industry has mobilized for war with a spreading epidemic of fat, we can't expect our government to stand in the way of health and longevity, nor mute for very long the fat sound of cash registers ringing up the sales.

However grave its issues may seem, the whole debate around dexfenfluramine may prove to be only a minor skirmish in the war against fat. New weapons are being added to the armamentarium with startling rapidity. Whether or not they prove to be the silver bullet that magically kills the monster fat remains to be seen. But these new discoveries seem to be attacking the problem of fat at its most fundamental genetic and biochemical basis. They promise new substances with the power to melt fat away, with no trouble and no adverse consequences.

There would seem to be a medical use for drugs that could reduce obesity in the morbidly obese. But the intense excitement on Wall Street that surrounds companies, like Interneuron, which make diet drugs has nothing to do with the plight of the morbidly obese. The traders know that 85 percent of the women in America, and in many places around the world, would pay any amount of money for the little pill that made the pounds of fat vanish before your eyes.

Let me be clear: I am no expert in these matters. I'm a French professor and a writer. I'm only a fat layman, who is interested in what is happening to fat in the world around me and on me. I'm no expert in the way diet drugs affect people's lives, but who is? The scientists and nutritionists working with pharmaceutical companies?—the ones who tell us the truth, only the truth about fat? Is it from them that we will learn whether the society should tolerate the administration of these drugs on a vast scale. Who can tell us how much these drugs will ever be used to accomplish actual benefits to health and how much they will just be bought greedily by women and men who want to look thin. Who can judge what the social cost might be of allowing these drugs to be used and misused? Who knows who the experts are?

Suppose we grant that it would be a boon to public health if everyone who wanted to be thin could get thin by taking a pill. At the very least it seems such a pill, with its effect on weight, would reduce the incidence of heart disease and cancer, if you believe widespread medical judgment. A question, nevertheless, arises. In order to stay thin, would you have to continue taking the pill? If you stopped, wouldn't you put the weight back on plus the usual additional premium that normally comes when you gain weight back after dieting?

So then, to stay thin, you would have to stay on the drug. But what would that mean for public health? Nobody can guess or gauge the effects of long-term drugs on a vast population. Prudent medical science would resist performing vast experiments. Prudent medicine would resist administering powerful drugs that transform the body's metabolism, its deepest cravings for food, in order to reduce even further small risks of early death. Particularly when doctors suspect that patients taking this drug are motivated as much by aesthetic as medical reasons!

Even newer diet drugs are on the horizon. Medically or chemically or genetically speaking, we are poised on the edge of a revolution. Witness the recent discovery of the so-called fat gene, and the miraculous hormone it manufactures: leptin. The body produces this natural substance, which tells the body when it is making too much fat. If administered to fat rats, they become thin; normal rats become anorexic. As if from heaven, out of our own bodies scientists will give us a substance that already tells the body when it's fat enough, which turns on the body's capacity to make fat. Leptin is the magic bullet, conceived by geneticists, who have been looking for the substance by which to banish our burden of fat once and for all.

There are many reasons why leptin may prove to be disappointing, as have so many magic bullets in the past. Nevertheless, its discovery in mice allows us for the first time to envision the possibility of a final fat finale—the fat lady singing it's over for fat. We now know that a magic bullet might exist, could exist, and, it seems like only a matter of time, will soon be among us. Maybe in this decade, maybe in thirty years, a final fat solution will be found. To my mind, postmodern fat becomes a cultural problem at this moment when, like the cigarette, it may be at the point of becoming extinct.

Things are moving very fast toward the full understanding of the genetic basis of fat. Early this year, the *New York Times* announced the discovery of another hormone, GLP-1, which acts like leptin to tell the brain that the body has eaten its fill.* Whereas

---

* *New York Times,* January 4, 1996.

leptin works over time to keep the body's fat supply stable, GLP-1 works instantly to give mice that bloated feeling, even after they've eaten only a couple of pellets. Scientists had already known that GLP-1 works in the stomach to slow absorption of protein so that the body can absorb sugar for instant energy. It also triggers the production of insulin in a gush, like what happens to the body after eating a big meal. Insulin, of course, helps the body break down glucose to make it available as energy for cells. But GLP-1 also works directly in the brain to send a signal that enough is enough. Scientists found that by blocking GLP-1 in rats, they kept on eating, getting fat, becoming diabetic. When they injected high quantities of GLP-1 into rat brains, thin and hungry rats started acting like they had just had Thanksgiving dinner.

GLP-1 is produced in the brain by the hypothalamus, the feeding control center. Scientists speculate that it is high levels of leptin, produced by fat cells, that signal the hypothalamus to produce GLP-1, which tells the rat it's full. Leptin attaches to receptors in the brain that may turn on a gene that directs the production of GLP-1 by the hypothalamus. If those leptin receptors are faulty, or pathways are blocked that lead from the receptors to the cells, then the brain will never get the message that the body's had enough fat already and eating will continue. Obesity may therefore be the result of leptin signals badly sent or ill received.

When scientists discovered that genetically obese rats got thin when they gave them leptin, they hoped that fat people were similarly deprived. No such luck. On the contrary, fat people have more leptin and more insulin than thin people; they just don't use it efficiently, or something. It's as if they were leptin resistant; even vast amounts of it don't seem to make any difference. The paradox, then, would be something like this: Your body contains a substance that keeps you thin, as long as you are thin. If you get fat, you have the same substance, in much larger quantities, but it doesn't work to affect your fat. So therefore, it follows, leptin given to thin people would work brilliantly to make them thinner, but wouldn't do anything at all for people who are fat.

Suppose fat disappears. What then? When scientists at last have made fat vanish, or, better yet, can control it, as in mice, within an inch of your hips, what then? At that moment, what will have been lost? Surely, disaster will have struck for a $30 billion business. All but one small segment of the diet industry will fold, all except the company that has the patent for human leptin, whatever, and permission to produce and market it. On that day, when our wishes will be granted, when fat at last will be in our grasp, in the grasp of our control, then we will learn how fickle fat fashion is, and how easily its taste can change. Have I got news for you?

Did you see those two adorable mice that appeared in the newspapers when the news of leptin was announced? The fat mouse and the thin mouse? Actually he's not thin, he's just normal looking compared to the fat one. The fat one, genetically obese, is pretty cute. One thing struck a lot of people about that picture of the fat mouse. They couldn't get over how cute he was, the fat one, compared to your regular, normally skinny mouse. I mean even if you didn't like mice, in general, you couldn't help but like this little guy, so fat and furry, with a cute round face that looks a lot more like Mickey Mouse than the pointy-nosed, skinny creature on his right. Cuteness is the quality that attaches to things that are small, immature, but cunningly devised. The fat mouse is much more adorable, more like a fat round baby, even if it's bigger and bulkier than the skinny, regular-size mouse. A BIG BABY is the most compelling thing in the world. P. T. Barnum understood that when for decades, at every circus stop, he would sponsor a contest to crown the most beautiful baby. The fattest one always won. Even today a family thrills when a big one is born. We want our babies big and fat and beautiful, when they're babies. Things, of course, change as early as two or three, when some kids, considered obese, begin to be treated as fatties. But the qualities that make a fat mouse cute, or a fat baby compelling, belong to old, deep strains of our aesthetic history, the history of what we find beautiful. It would take very little for them to re-emerge as the energetic source of a whole new taste in fashion, an abrupt return to loving fat. At the very moment, when fat is about to disappear under the onslaught of genetic engineering and fundamental understanding of its production—at that very moment, fashion, I'll bet, will reverse. When everyone can be thin by popping a pill, suddenly fat will look hot. It may have already started to happen; all around us the first faint signs of a fat revolution on its way are beginning dimly to be perceived. We can state it as an inflexible rule: The faster the diet industry learns to eliminate fat, the closer we get to a shift in taste, when fat again will be beautiful. When that day comes, the diet industry, quick to adjust, will shift gears and begin digging up old copies of T. C. Duncan's classic, *How to Become Plump*, written less than a hundred years ago.*

---

* T. C. Duncan, *How to Become Plump, or Talks on Physiological Feeding* (Chicago: Duncan Brothers, 1878).

In the meantime, we have been given Olestra, a synthetic fat molecule that passes through the gastrointestinal tract without being absorbed. It isn't a fat substitute, like many that are already on the market; it *is* fat, with the same power to make food taste good, to soothe the palate with its creamy smoothness on the tongue. (In addition, it has a slight aftertaste.)

The FDA has just approved the use and marketing of Olestra. We may very soon, perhaps already, be able to eat fat-free fat in potato chips or French fries, or even at Thanksgiving dinner. On the one hand, it will save lives, it's claimed, by reducing the fat in diets, and the consequent risks of heart disease, diabetes, and some cancers. On the other hand, Olestra has a few problems. According to *Time* magazine, "It can trigger intestinal cramping, flatulence and loose bowels."[*] Not only loose, but running and dripping, since in some people the stuff promotes what is delicately called "fecal urgency," and "anal leakage." More important, Olestra inhibits the body from absorbing certain essential nutrients, like vitamins A, D, E, K, and especially beta-carotene, a valuable anti-oxidant, which may discourage certain cancers. The FDA has presumably weighed the eventual health advantages against the risks and inconveniences Olestra represents. Unlike diet drugs, this is a food additive, which millions of people may well begin eating every day in enormous quantities, persuaded that it's somehow better for their health, and more likely to ensure the elusive goal of thin. Distributed over a whole population, one consumed by the need to cut fat, who knows what consequences

[*] *Time,* January 8, 1996.

for public health its widespread introduction into our diets may have?

But even if it works, even if scientists find a way to eliminate its harmful effects, will Olestra work to make us thin? Don't bet on it. Nabisco's SnackWell's cookies are fat free, but they've still got plenty of calories. According to Thomas Hoban, a professor of sociology and food science at North Carolina State University, "people have a tendency to eat a lot more of them."[*] Just as Americans have grown increasingly obese by consuming more and more low-fat, no-fat, and fat-free food, so we're likely to really bulk up once we start eating Olestra—well, not exactly Olestra, but what surrounds it. *Time* magazine has pictures of a deep, rich-looking slice of peach pie, which ordinarily has 405 calories. Made with Olestra, the same slice looks as good, but it has only 252 calories. It looks so good you could eat a couple of those puppies, at the risk of anal leak, and get just as fat or fatter as you would by eating real fat. Who among us won't be tempted to slice a little bigger piece, or have an extra helping, when it's only half the calories and the fat we crave is fat-free?

Dr. Ornish encourages you to eat complex carbohydrates: "The Reversal diet consists primarily of *complex carbohydrates*, also known as starches."[†] No one would discount the benefits to people with heart disease, with arteriosclerosis, to be derived from eating the sort of radically low-fat diet Dr. Ornish prescribes. As he writes,

[*] Ibid.

[†] Dean Ornish, M.D., *Dr. Dean Ornish's Program for Reversing Heart Disease* (New York: Ballantine Books, 1990), p. 257.

"No one in the Framingham study ever had a heart attack whose total blood cholesterol was less than 150."[*] Assume his diet protects the diseased from heart attacks, as he claims, but does it also insure them, or us, against other diseases to which humans today are commonly liable?

Consider olive oil. Dr. Ornish is no fan. He writes, "Olive oil, for example, contains 1.9 grams of saturated fat per tablespoon (about 14 percent saturated fat). So if you add olive oil to your food, you are adding saturated fat to your food—and the more you add, the more your cholesterol level will increase. . . . In other words, olive oil and safflower oil are not 'good' for you; they are less 'bad' for you."[†]

Conversely, in the *New York Times*, Jane Brody reported that, in a study by Dr. Dimitrios Trichopoulos at Harvard, "American women might actually experience as much as a 50 percent reduction in breast cancer risk if they consumed more olive oil."[‡] So what do you say, what do you do? Do you eat more olive oil or less? That's the question. And what about salt, usually a no-no? Dr. Ornish demurs, "If you don't have high blood pressure, then you don't have to limit your salt intake drastically."[§]

Dr. Ornish aims, of course, to cut your cholesterol. But how dangerous is it? It depends. The *New York Times* reported that "Cholesterol levels, which so accurately predict risk of heart disease

[*] Ibid., p. 268.
[†] Ornish, p. 265.
[‡] Jane Brody, "New Evidence on the Benefits of Olive Oil," *New York Times*, January 18, 1995.
[§] Ornish, p. 271.

in middle-aged people, appear to have no such predictive value in the elderly."[*] Dr. Stephen B. Hulley, chairman of the department of epidemiology and biostatistics at the University of California, San Francisco, is quoted saying his study shows that people after the age of seventy "can take it easy and relax" and stop worrying about cholesterol. Taking it easy, relaxing, and not worrying about cholesterol may in general be better for your health than anything you can do to diminish cholesterol, he thinks. Dr. Hulley said he was "deeply concerned because many people in their late 70's and older were taking" cholesterol-lowering drugs. It's hard to predict what long-term effects anti-cholesterol drugs may have. Taking Niacin, of course, has potential side effects on the liver. Other anti-cholesterol drugs can pose dangers as well. Besides, it's not exactly the amount of cholesterol that matters; high cholesterol isn't so bad if your so-called good cholesterol isn't low, and low good cholesterol may not be bad if your bad cholesterol isn't high. It's the ratio of bad to good, doctors think, that increases the risk of heart attacks.

Low-fat diets, like those of Dr. Ornish, eliminate animal protein. "The protein that comes from eating a T-bone steak is exactly the same quality as the protein that comes from a meal of rice and beans," he writes. "But when you eat a steak, you're also consuming excessive saturated fat and cholesterol."[†] Yet eating mostly starches has its own health risks, and has been discouraged on the editorial page of the *New York Times*. In a headline the paper thunders, "*Basta* With the Pasta," and the editors continue, "According to

[*] *New York Times,* October 2, 1994.
[†] Ornish, p. 260.

assorted weight-loss experts and obesity researchers (a.k.a. 'spoil-sports'), a high-carbohydrate regimen—i.e., starchy stuff like pasta and bread—may be inappropriate for the insulin-resistant, who constitute at least 25 percent of all Americans, and for the over-weight, who are about 33 percent of us."[*]

In fact, *pace* Dr. Ornish, there are those like Richard Heller, Ph.D., and Rachael Heller, Ph.D., both of New York's Mount Sinai School of Medicine, who, in their article "Healthy for Life," encourage people to eat bacon, sausage, and pastrami, which they call "risk reducing foods," arguing that since they are carbohydrate free they reduce production of insulin and hence discourage the accumulation of fat.[†] Insulin turns glucose into fat. Those who are insulin resistant secrete excess insulin, especially when they eat a lot of carbohydrates, turning more of it into fat. Hence, such people ought to eat more protein and fat, which is low in carbohydrates.

In a similar vein, Gerald Reaven, M.D., of the Stanford University School of Medicine, argues against the claims of Dr. Ornish that "there's nothing magical about low-fat that makes you lose weight." He means that if you take in fewer calories from fats but add back as many in the form of pasta and other low- or non-fat foods, you won't shed pounds. He thinks that "the call to replace fats in the diet with starches and other carbohydrates can be contributing to heart disease in a significant proportion of the population"—that is, in those who are insulin resistant, who turn carbohydrates into fat, raising cholesterol levels—mainly the ratio of

[*] *New York Times,* January 24, 1996.
[†] *Tufts University Diet and Nutrition Letter* 13, no. 3 (1995): 5.

bad to good. Dr. Ornish's Reversal diet is 10 percent fat, 70–75 percent carbohydrate. According to Dr. Reaven, that could kill you. He thinks that for the insulin resistant, you ought to be doing 45 percent carbohydrates and 40 percent fat, "since fat does not lead to an increase in insulin secretion."[*]

The *New York Times* ran a lengthy story on the latest diet guru, Dr. Stephen Gullo.[†] Well-known clients like Donald Trump, Anna Sui, and Princess Yasmin Khan, pay $500 for the initial interview and $175 for weekly twenty-minute sessions to get the benefit of his diet pep talks and exuberant, exclamatory advice. The rest of us can read his book, whose title, flying in the face of all experience, proclaims *Thin Tastes Better.* Dr. Gullo, the year's diet star, may be perceived to be advocating the anti-Ornish diet. What the *New York Times* calls his "retro" diet, high in protein and low in carbohydrates, is a throwback, no doubt, to the earliest published diets. According to Hillel Schwartz, Mr. William Banting, a fashionable London undertaker, proposed in 1863 the first extensive published diet, featuring lean meat, dry toast, soft-boiled eggs, and green vegetables. With it, "Banting" became, as Schwartz says "the new participle for reducing" in this century.[‡] According to Gullo, recommending pasta and bread and potatoes, the recent low-fat alternative, is "dietary Disneyland." According to him, the high-starch diets not only produce insulin and hence more fat in the insulin

[*] *New York Times,* April 26, 1995.

[†] Ibid.

[‡] Hillel Schwartz, *Never Satisfied: A Cultural History of Diets, Fantasies, and Fat* (New York: Free Press, 1986), p. 101.

resistant, they encourage people's tendency to binge by stimulating their appetites. He dismisses recent evidence that obesity may be genetically determined. "Genes," he says, "may set the lower limit, but you set the upper limit."

Dr. Gullo is the hero of another article in the *Times,* one devoted to what is called responsible eating.* Dr. Gullo advises his rich and famous clients on how to eat frugally in the temples of gastronomy, where their wealth and power oblige them to dine on all too frequent occasions. The clients require the advice of Dr. Gullo on how to avoid the alluring temptations of fabulous fat served up beautifully or calling to them from menus at, say, La Grenouille in New York or at Bouley's. It isn't easy to "watch" what you eat, in a three-star restaurant, if watching means not eating, as it usually does. Who wants to look but not eat—at those prices?

Dr. Gullo has a diet philosophy that seems perfectly attuned to the worldview of his high-rolling clients. "Bodies have budgets like a business does. You want to spend calories the way you do money." Calories are money; eating is spending. So Dr. Gullo goes to the most expensive restaurants in New York and spends lots of real money, treating his food like virtual money not to be spent. He has this bizarre idea that when you go to Bouley's and they bring you a basket of their incredible rolls (the raisin ones and the thyme), the food scrooge waves them away. "That roll has two hundred twenty-five to three hundred calories without any butter," says Dr. Gullo. Say no to rolls. Say no to filet, to veal dishes, and cheese soufflé, say no to platters of chocolate and meringue Concorde, caramel custard, mixed

* *New York Times,* May 28, 1995.

berry tarts and Napoleons. It's not money the rich are afraid to spend, but calories, which are worth more than money. Calories have become more precious than money because money for these people is all but unlimited, whereas none of them dying to be thin has calories to spare. Dr. Gullo's practice confirms what we have already seen, that dieting is the most perfected form of consumption under conditions of advanced capitalism, ensuring the greatest amount of business for everyone all around. Dr. Gullo makes out, Daniel Bouley makes out, and the dieter leaves the restaurant unsatisfied, dreaming of another expensive meal. And someone gets to eat those rolls.

This book starts from the premise that dieting makes you fat, and the machine for gaining weight is the yo-yo. Lose some, gain it back in spades, lose some more, and grow fatter. The fat-acceptance movement has for a long time pointed to the baleful effects of yo-yo dieting: a decreased rate at which the body burns calories; more fat and less muscle tissue; more difficulty losing weight the next time; increased risk for heart disease and diabetes; even premature death. But a new report, issued by the National Task Force on the Prevention and Treatment of Obesity is meant to be reassuring: "There is no convincing evidence that weight cycling adversely affects health."* The conclusion of the task force is puzzling. They discounted evidence that wrestlers who yo-yo dieted "to make weight" had significantly lower metabolic rates than non-yo-yoing wrestlers. That would mean that, over time, yo-yo dieting puts the body's metabolism at a disadvantage so far as future dieting is concerned. Each subsequent diet will be less effective at reduc-

* *Tufts University Diet and Nutrition Letter* 12, no. 10 (December 1994): 3.

ing the would-be dieter's weight. The body's previous experiences with diets will have trained it to store fat more easily and to offer greater resistance to attempts to eliminate its replenished stores of fat.

Kelly Brownell, Ph.D., professor of psychology and director of the Yale Center for Eating and Weight Disorders in New Haven, is one of those who resists the notion that diets don't work, that obesity results from dieting, which in turn causes most eating disorders. The truth is, says Dr. Brownell, that "people *have* dieted down and kept it off."° She says a lot of them are just not accounted for because they do it on their own, rather than participating in clinical studies. Maybe that means that the really successful dieters are the ones the doctors never see, since the vast majority of those regain all their lost weight after three or four years. Maybe going to a doctor to lose weight guarantees that you won't succeed. Maybe doctors cause fat.

Dr. Brownell's own view is "that sometimes drastic things work. I don't want to rule out any approaches."† Even though drastic approaches mostly fail, she's ready to try anything. In a piece appearing on the Op-Ed page of the *New York Times* entitled "Get Slim With Higher Taxes."‡ Dr. Brownell deplores the fact that "while the Government has imposed so-called sin taxes on cigarettes and alcohol in order to reduce consumption, it has yet to consider taxing low-nutrition food or banning commercials for fatty snacks targeted at children." She goes on to make the following alarming, political sug-

° *Tufts University Diet and Nutrition Letter* 12, no. 8 (October 1994): 6.
† Ibid.
‡ *New York Times,* December 15, 1995.

gestions: "Congress and state legislatures could shift the focus to the environment [away from genetics] by taxing foods with little nutritional value. Fatty foods would be judged on their nutritive value per calorie or gram of fat; the least healthy would be given the highest tax rate. Consumption of high-fat food would drop, and the revenue could be used for public exercise facilities—bike paths and running tracks—or nutrition education in schools."

To the already bloated bureaucracy, Dr. Brownell would add a fat czar. With the best intentions in the world, the Yale nutritionist would make the fat pay sin taxes for their pleasures, raising monies to be used to finance the activities of the thin. The thin, who already are likely to be the rich, would get another tax break; the poor, likely to be fat, would be the object of the government's tough love. Dr. Brownell, who often speaks sensibly about fat, has gone over the edge with this proposal, which I take to be serious. So persuaded is he of the evil of fat, so convinced that we must combat it at all cost, that he is prepared to mobilize the government in a war on fat. Like the war on drugs, this one is likely to be waged at immense social cost and with no greater likelihood of success. This latest proposal seems rather like the logical outcome of the whole current wave of anti-fat propaganda, raised to an even more hysterical pitch and leading to even scarier demands for action. In the minds of these well-meaning scientists, fat is such a danger to the body politic that it warrants further governmental intrusions into people's lives, and additional confiscation of their wealth. Nowhere in all this talk of taxing fat food do we hear a single good word for the blessing of chocolate, the balm of chicken soup, or the comfort of a nicely schmeared bagel.

Part Three

THE
CONCEPT *FAT*

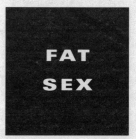

FAT
SEX

The following statement of purpose appeared on the masthead of the first issue of *Fat Girl*[*]: "*Fat Girl* is a zine for and about Fat Dykes. *Fat Girl* seeks to create a broad-based dialogue that both challenges and informs our notion of Fat-Dyke-identity." It hasn't been widely known until now that there even was such a thing as a Fat-Dyke identity, or that it needed to be challenged and informed by a "broad-based" dialogue. Anyway, what exactly does broad-based mean here? Is that insulting word for women, as in "dumb broad," being taken back here, reversed in value, and turned around against the male oppressors who fling it? Just as calling a big woman "fat girl" would be an insult, except when it's used affec-

---

[*] *Fat Girl* (San Francisco: Fat Girl Publishing, 1994).

tionately, admiringly, by someone positively assuming and bravely affirming their identity. So maybe a broad-based dialogue is one reserved for fat broads.

But it probably means something else. The statement on the *Fat Girl* masthead continues, "We come in all shapes and sizes; from diverse ethnic cultures and different class backgrounds." So it also indicates that there is a diversity of voices speaking here, from the standpoint of many different perspectives, who at bottom participate in the same broadly shared identity.

But broad-based may also mean big butts. There's an ad for a computer program, CoSession for Windows (Triton Technologies); it features three big fat guys, seen from behind, sitting at a counter in a diner. All three have enormous behinds, and pants sliding down revealing a horizontal expanse of skin between belt and shirt, and just the top of the crack in their ass—a hint of décolleté derrière. The headline says, "The Fastest. No Buts About It." And the copy begins. "These guys are going nowhere fast. So they may not care that CoSession for Windows is the fastest remote control software." The reader who sent the ad to *Bulk Male*, a magazine for gay fat men and those who love them, writes, "I found this ad in one of my computer magazines and thought you would get a chuckle out of it. I would have loved to have been the photographer." The photographer probably thought those fat asses made a funny picture. Certainly the fat-phobic creators of the ad thought so and thought readers would too. What is surely true is that the picture gives a new meaning to the phrase "a broad-based dialogue."

The joke here is on the photographer who thought that this image of three large fat butts lined up like that could only be a hoot. But to readers of *Bulk Male,* this is no joke, and that's funny. That's why the letter writer sends this ad to the editors, who, he thinks, will find it funny but no joke either. Lovers of fat asses like them, like the reader, get a chuckle from having the last laugh, from laughing at the laughter of fat-phobes, who don't even realize they are printing a rare, and thus particularly arousing, kind of pornography in a computer magazine. What the photographer and the ad-makers thought was funny, the reader thinks is hot. He would have loved to be that photographer, to gaze rapturously, excitedly, at those mounds of broad-based flesh, and to shoot. For him, those fat butts, supposed to be sexless, going nowhere fast, are quick and dirty, nasty, pornographic. He gets off on what looks funny to others and disdains their disdain, 'cause they don't get it. The fat-phobes, who think these fat guys are going nowhere, would probably be astounded to think that anyone could get off on this ad. They wouldn't dream that someone might actually masturbate to this and cut this picture out of a computer magazine because it turned him on. It comes as a shock whenever you realize that what you take for granted as being ugly or funny is beautiful or sexy in the eyes of someone else. Some of this material is pornographic, in that it explicitly aims to excite FAs (fat-admirers), readers and viewers, to masturbate. But most of it is merely obscene, making nakedly visible what we have come to expect will stay permanently out of sight.

It is amazing still, in America, to listen to people tell you how much they hate the sight of fat. Look at the face of a woman as it scrunches up at the thought or sight of fat, on herself or on some-one else. But reading these magazines, we hear other voices, the dreams and hungers of people who love fat and find it beautiful. And, I'll say it again, loving beautiful fat has been the rule, not the exception, in human history, and one day it will rule again.

Or get this.

Here's a passage from a letter sent to the editors of *Fat Girl*, which they chose to publish in the second issue. The enthusiastic correspondent writes, "I think my favorite part of the first issue were the photos of women feeding each other. So pornographic!!!! I don't think I've ever seen pictures of big women eating, happily eating, much less feeding each other with such obvious enjoyment. Those pictures just shot an electric current through me."

What is it about that that looks good, excites her, and makes her happy? How come I've never before seen pictures of fat women eating? Much less feeding each other?

Gael Greene in *Blue Skies No Candy* keeps on deliciously rewriting the same sex scene, where someone's eating food off someone else's body—good food, good body.* A lot of the pictures in *Fat Girl* or in *Bulk Male* are about flesh and food, bringing sex into close erotic connection with eating, illustrating intensely mouthy pleasures of lapping, licking, slurping, gulping, blowing, sucking, bolting, blubbering. Eating greedily, copiously in public, eating rich foods avidly out of hands or off the body of someone feeding you, these are pleasures many of us can barely allow ourselves to contemplate. For most people, feeding—the act of eating and food—has become such a highly charged issue that they obscure it with privacy, surround it with precautions and taboos, never do it exuberantly or only in the deepest secret.

Fat people eating in public, eating in full view of others, violates some taboo. Most fat people do most of their serious eating

---

* Gael Greene, *Blue Skies, No Candy* (New York: Morrow, 1976).

out of sight. At the table, they don't appear to be eating any more than anyone else. Many fat people, in fact, are normal eaters, with metabolisms that make them fat. But a lot of fat people, like many thin and all bulimic ones, binge. You rarely see them eat abnormally at the table. But you know that a lot of eating is going on out of the public eye. To be seen eating a lot, to be fat and be seen eating at all, makes you look like a pig. Pigs are repulsive or funny at best.

Fat makes a lot of people laugh. Why? It is not that the fat are happy; the more laughter they provoke the gloomier they get. It's that the very appearance of fat, the fact of fat, reveals what is supposed to be the dirty little secret, the moral failing: that the bearer or wearer of fat indulges a compulsive drive to eat that's out of control. If that's true, and it probably isn't, it's probably not the eating that made you fat; it's the guilt and shame of being fat that makes you eat. Most of us can hide our vices, if we choose to. Not the fat. Their fat speaks up, speaks loudly, about what is most important in their life, the minute they walk in a room. That's why fat people spend their lives creating lies about their eating, hiding the moments of bulimia or of repeated, decisive sneaking. Marlon Brando had a big lock put on his refrigerator to keep himself from bingeing at night, then secretly ordered food out, which had to be thrown to him over the wall.

I thought about my mother's cousin Molly. They went for years to spas. They lost thousands of pounds at great expense. I asked my mother how they got so fat. It wasn't simply genetic, she said.

You take Molly. Her father was a "big" man, but her mother wasn't. But Molly was a sneaky eater.

What do you mean, Mom?

She always had candy handy.

And as she said that, "candy handy," she made a gesture with her hand like a gambler scooping up dice. A gesture of urgent appropriation, making yours what no one else at that moment can have. It's mine, this handful of chocolate, and no one is going to interrupt the elegant but powerful gesture with which I take another turn, my turn, my hand at this sure pleasure. This is a pleasure I can enjoy and enjoy, being sure in advance of enjoying, since it's always at hand.

Do you think there are a lot of fat people like Molly who sneak food?

I think most. They want people to think it's genetic.

But why does she have to sneak it, Ma? What would happen if anyone saw?

They'd think she was a pig,

What's a pig, Ma?

A pig is someone who eats when they aren't hungry.

Why do they do that?

For the pure pleasure of it.

But they're sneaking their pleasure. Maybe they get pleasure from the sneaking?

No, I don't think so.

But, there's gotta be a lot of guilt.

Oh! yes, lottsa guilt.

So the pure pleasure of eating without hunger, without need, eating only for taste and well-being, comes accompanied with the cruel inbite of remorse. The pleasure is not pure at all; your conscience is bitten by what you bite. Every time you take that moment out of your day to sink your teeth into the brilliant darkness of a rich

Belgian chocolate, or touch your tongue to the pleasing, yielding hardness of a chocolate Snickers bar, that moment of intense pleasure provokes instantly a pang, a shiver of guilt, and a sense of deeper anxiety at postponing the moment of definitive reform. Because one cannot live one's life feeling in the eyes of the world like a pig.

Poor pig! Little pigs, we know, are like babies, smart, lovable, silly animals very close to children. Pigs make you laugh because they cannot stop eating whatever slop you put in front of them. An automatic compulsion, a mechanical repetition, seems to control the pig, and at that moment, for all their resemblance, they are something less than human: little eating machines. We observe them. We observe the distance between their ridiculous shape and our own more or less normal one, and we feel superior; at the same time we nervously estimate the not infinite distance between us and them, the troubling connection we feel between their visible compulsion and our hidden one. Laughter at fat is a compromise between fear that we may be just like those pigs and the fleeting assurance that, at least in our mind's eye, we aren't.

One thing, Ma. Do you imagine that your family doesn't know, more or less exactly, how and when you sneak chocolate?

Of course, I think they don't know!

We know she knows that we know she sneaks around. In families, much is hidden but there are no secrets. Everyone knows what is going on all the time, even if at first or even at last they pretend they don't. Probably no one keeps a secret from his or her family very long, unless everyone agrees that it should be kept. The sneaking doesn't fool anyone; it's just a way of acknowledging to yourself that a taboo is being violated, that what you're doing ought not to come to light. Maybe the first or second time, you hide to keep yourself from being punished for the little transgression you're about to commit. But pretty soon, hiding becomes indispensable to the pleasure. Hiding gives the eating that little electric current that makes it exciting, erotic, intense. Hiding intensifies the pleasure with intimations of danger, risk and interdiction. After a while you can get to the point where you don't know anymore what you love more, the sneaking or the chocolates. Since the world is getting generally fatter (except for some famines), more and more of our eating is probably being done out of sight.

There's a real sense of transgressing taboos in the spectacle of those women giving each other things to eat, to suck and lick. The rule of this benign sort of S/M says that the eater can't touch what the feeder gives her to eat. Pieces of fudge are pushed into her mouth, she's forced to suck or slurp long, slender popsicles, toes are shoved onto her tongue, she's made to gob wads of whipped cream piled on tips of heavy clodded shoes, little bunches of grapes are dropped into her waiting throat, cannelloni are stuffed in whole, big pieces of cake dripping with icing, éclairs eaten sideways, a piece of chocolate so big it takes two hands, an enormous tit, a vast chubby belly that she has to suck and kiss and slide her mouth along.

The reader writing to the editor doesn't think she's ever seen this before, pictures of fat women eating—not only eating but happily feeding, eating with such obvious relish. To be able to look at that spectacle turns her on. The taboo that makes fat funny makes it perversely, powerfully erotic when the taboo is transgressed, when you let yourself enjoy what you are supposed to hate and fear.

One might wonder if fat-admirers, living in a time of fat phobia, love fat with anything like the pure immediacy, the spontaneous sentiment with which people living in fat-philiac times do. How much of the erotic attraction to fat women is a function of the disapproval or revulsion with which they are normally seen. Does the sexiness come from the perversion of what is supposed to be normal—from loving something abnormal? In a fat utopia, will a magazine like *Fat Girl* need to exist? Will there be any reason to publish it, when fat is generally seen to be beautiful?

In the first "Fat Girl Round Table," the conversation gets around to body-image talk. Selena, who looks like she's close to 250 pounds, doesn't want to have to hear that fat is beautiful. She doesn't want her lover, who is smaller than she, telling her what big beautiful juicy tits she has. She doesn't want men who love fat women to tell her how they love her big fat ass and get off on the rolls of fat that flow down the sides of her stomach.

Selena doesn't want praise for being fat, because she doesn't trust it. She can't trust this praise; it's probably fat-phobic. If you're having constantly to talk about how beautiful fat is, you're probably trying to talk yourself into something. You probably feel fat-averse and are working out your problem with a fatty. Selena doesn't need you to work out your fat phobia with her. Nor does April Miller, who says, "I've had very brief relationships with people who have this bizarre . . . fascinated/repulsed kind of thing going on."[*]

Imagine the complexity of feelings when you're really fat, and you find yourself to be the object of the fascinated attention of someone who is thin. And then think how it hurts when you realize that the fascination—the excited curiosity and appreciation of your fat—arises out of some deep revulsion. Naturally, such relation-

---

[*] *Fat Girl*, p. 38.

ships are brief. The fat woman immediately starts to feel like her fat is exotic, like some rare bird, desirable only because unfamiliar, a beautiful ugliness, an alluring freak. It's the same discomfort that arises when whites take to praising the tawny beauty of blacks. The fascination is the form that a certain repulsion assumes in order to conceal its fear.

So on the one hand, the fat woman who hears her beauty praised has to wonder if it isn't the language of someone deeply averse to her fat. But on the other, she also has to fear the opposite. That this person who is praising her beauty is a chubby chaser, a pervert who is interested in her exclusively for her fat. Such a pervert has no care at all for the person in the fat, only for the surface flesh and its abundance. It's only the body they want, not the soul of fat. These dykes are suspicious not only of men, but of chubby-chasing dykes, who have their own fears and hatred of fat, which they enact in the form of a perverse fascination and compulsive enthusiasm for it.

Chubby chasers are viewed with suspicion not only because they are considered perverts. In the case of men who chase fat women, their interest is suspected of betraying a convulsive desire to control. Some thin men are aware that there are fat women whose desperation and low self-esteem cause them to throw themselves at skinny men who show them any interest. April Miller stopped going to NAAFA conventions because she was always getting the vibes that told her these men wanted women who were desperate and powerless. The guys get to be like gods to fat women ready and sadly eager at any cost to make themselves available to what they fear they may never deserve, thin men.

A lot of men who love fat women complain about these women's low self-esteem, which makes them so suspicious of any thin man who loves them. Many of these guys insist that their attraction to these women arises naturally, out of the admiration they have always felt for the fleshy beauty of abundant size. They resent being considered perverts by women whose fat they admire.

In his memoirs, *Real Women Don't Diet*, Ken Mayer writes how hard it was as an adolescent, growing up in love with fat girls: "I definitely prefer the heavier ones, because the skinny ones look so frail and insignificant. I can't decide which is more confusing, that my friends prefer thinner girlfriends than I do, or that they question my choices."*

I keep coming back to Selena, who doesn't want to hear any of this fat women's body talk. Probably not from Ken Mayer, probably not from me. Who is to say that this book itself doesn't arise out of the fascination/repulsion she describes and abhors? That's the risk I have to run. I don't love all fat, but I love a lot of it. I don't love much skinny, but it has turned me on. This is not a book that aims to promote fat acceptance, but it doesn't want to contribute to fat aversion. On the contrary, it respects the political movement for fat acceptance. Under the present regime of body fashion, given the suffering to which the fat have been subjected, and the disdain they continue to endure, fat is a political, is a feminist issue. But this book is not political in any effectively real sense. It is, rather,

---

* Ken Mayer, *Real Women Don't Diet: One Man's Praise of Large Women and His Outrage at the Society That Rejects Them* (Silver Spring, Md.: Bartleby Press, 1993), p. 23.

utopian. It is trying to see fat from the perspective of its having been and once again becoming beautiful. It tries to recall the past in order to anticipate the future when fat again will be fine, will be fabulous and fair, brilliant, chic, smart, and phat. I happen to think that time is coming soon, very soon. We are living these days on the cusp of a radical transformation of the way our eyes see beauty. Hillel Schwartz predicted the same thing over ten years ago. He was wrong then. The taste in thin has grown only stronger. I could be wrong; I've been wrong before.

But even if I'm wrong and the revolution in taste is long in coming, one thing is sure. It will come. There will come a day when fat

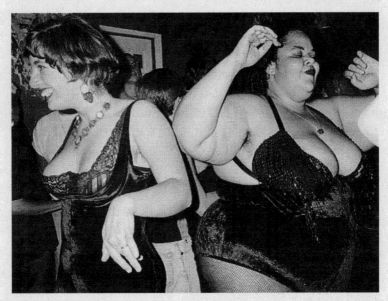

Revi and April

will be beautiful and skinny will be hated and feared, as it always has been. Nearly always has been. Except for a few brief moments in human history, fat is what felt beautiful. It is not this book's intention to be political, to persuade or exhort or encourage. It aims to be prophetic, to imagine from the perspective of the present the horizon of a time when fat forms flower.

To transvalue the value of fat is a process to which this book may contribute, but which is probably inevitable anyway, ineluctable, irresistible. As the wheel of body fashion slowly turns, as new conditions arise that make fat desirable, our looks and the way we look at fat will change.

The zine *Fat Girl* may be a harbinger of the revolution. It is the product of a cooperative, of women working together to give social value to what is seen to be hateful, to appreciate what is devalued and demeaned. It is hard work changing the way you see yourself in the mirror, when your image reflects only what is universally disapproved and despised. For these women it is constantly a struggle to learn to love what they hate. Bravely, they acknowledge the difficulty. Deva, the fat bottom whose skinny top is Laura, admits, despite her fat politics, that she struggles all the time.

> When you grow up fat and you're always fat and you've always been fat, you learn to ignore so much. You learn to deal with it. I have this wall, and most fat women I know do. You have to, or you would just cry all the time! You couldn't take that much hostility. It's a struggle to maintain your self-esteem.[*]

[*] *Fat Girl*, no. 3 (1995), p. 30.

The hostility others direct against the fat is so deeply internalized that fat people do the work of others on themselves. Self-hatred is what one hears in a great deal of the rhetoric of fat acceptance. But how, in our society, could one hear anything else, given the ferocity of the hostility directed against fat?

Max, a 300-pound lesbian, talked about the resentment that infects even the fat cooperative. She confesses, with some difficulty and shame, how hard she found it to accept others as being fat who were 100 pounds thinner than she. Her experience of being super-fat seemed to her to be of a whole other order of magnitude, and hence of a whole other quality, than that of women who happened to weigh in the neighborhood of only 200 pounds. For Max, one of the founders of *Fat Girl*, her identity as a fat woman is so tied to the pain she felt that she cannot allow others, less heavy than she, to share in her sense of liberation from self-hate. "If women much smaller than me are fat, what does that make me?"* Her identity politics, her fat identity, requires that she be able to identify what is authentically fat. But who knows what being fat means? If 200 pounds can seem thin to Max, then how can gaining seven or eight pounds seem fat to someone who is thin. In relation to our ideal weight we are all mostly fat. At what weight do we truly become oppressed in this society, severely disadvantaged not only in our own eyes but in the eyes of others by being fat? As with most liberation movements, which are about overcoming oppression, there is a sort of snobbism of suffering, in which those who are the most oppressed have the greatest moral claim on liberation. Your self-

---

* *Fat Girl*, no. 1 (1994), p. 18.

love, your whole sense of identity, depends on having had to overcome more suffering, more hostility and self-hate, than others have, who are almost as fat. Loving fat, surrounded by a world that hates it, is never easy, innocent, spontaneous, or fully free.*

On facing pages in *Fat Girl* are answers elicited from the community to two questions: What do you dislike about being fat, what do you like about it?† A lot of what these people like about being fat is a reaction to the way it is disliked, particularly on women. It's hard to know, if the world turned, if fat became generally beautiful, whether one would love one's fat for the same reasons these women have come to love it now when it's hated.

"I like my size!!!! I feel powerful and immovable."‡

Most women have been taught to take up less space, to shrink and slim down. These women like the sense of being substantial, being more dense, immovable, of assuming more space in the world. Mass and volume feel like power, reinforcing the strength of your social presence. The women are less intimidated, particularly by men. They impose themselves on social space by occupying more of it.

"I'm soft. When I give my body to someone I'm giving a lot."

Fat is generous, like a woman may be who is generously endowed. It is a a gift and it promotes giving. Beautiful fat breasts have the generosity of melons, call them cantaloupes, in which one wants to plunge one's face to drink in the freshness of so

* Ibid., p. 18.
† *Fat Girl,* no. 3 (1995), pp. 40–41.
‡ Ibid., p. 41.

much delicious flesh. Being fat makes you cuddly and warm; giving yourself to lovers, you give a lot of love, a lot of enfolding, embraceable flesh. Your fat body encircles, protects, comforts, and warms. It is a soft pillow onto which lovers sink and lose themselves in ease.

Perhaps it is time we thought more about what Eve Kosovsky Sedgwick calls, in a poem, "The Uses of Being Fat." She's a poetess of fatness, the inventor of fat criticism, a leader in the study of the way culture represents fat. She writes,*

> I used to have a superstition that
> there was this use to being fat:
> no one I loved could come to harm
> enfolded in my touch—
> that lots of me would blot it up,
> the rattling chill, night sweat or terror. . . .

Fat pillows. It enfolds, and protects, and gives love; it smothers with love and that's the problem but also the use of fat. It surrounds the one you love, like the magic circle of an amulet, and absorbs like a blotter the blows of the world; that, at least, is what you superstitiously like to think. In fact, the poem goes on to say, fat love tends to suffocate as much as it protects. Instead of comfort it causes those caught, drowned in its embrace to flee to places ever deeper inside themselves to escape the voracious embrace. There, turned

---

* *Fat Art, Thin Art* (Durham, N.C.: Duke University Press, 1994), p. 15

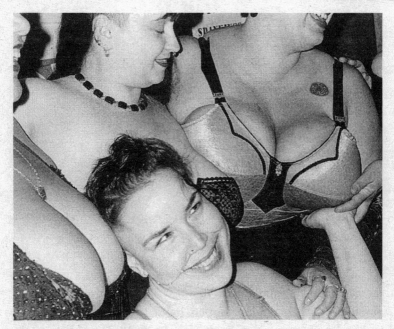

Devra in the sea of breasts

away from the enfolding touch, they discover not more ease but the greater horrors of loneliness and death. Still, the poet says, some truth may cling to the superstition. Maybe her embrace and the suffocating protection of fat love drive you deeper into places where, to avoid smothering, you learn to be more independent, tough-minded, and self-responsible. In a way, she says, fat love protects by overprotecting, making you flee its embrace, more determined to stand alone.

Another poet won't be caught in the trap of being cuddly. C. M. Donald writes,

TO THOSE WOMEN

To those women
Who find me cuddly,
Who like fat women
And want to hug them all:

I am not your mother,
Your baby or your shelter
And I am not your blasted teddy bear.°

This states pretty clearly, and with admirable poise, the difficult position one faces in trying to define and uphold, as well as challenge and inform, a fat dyke identity. Those women whose love she doesn't want are those who love all fat women, "and want to hug them all." I may be fat and cuddly, motherly and warm, protective, enfolding, but it is not just for that, indiscriminately, that I want to be loved; I am so much more than my fat. C. M. Donald illustrates here what I call the chubby dilemma. With one hand, you struggle to acquire a fat dyke identity, with the other you resist being loved for your identity alone.

One of the fat girls who answered the question "What do you like about being fat?" said this: "I like my fat. I like being large, powerful, sensuous, heavy, sexy, intimidating, inviting, enfolding, warm, extremely soft, able to stare down big creeps, able to take up a lot of room and annoy people, able to be a tender pillow for a sad

° C. M. Donald, *The Fat Woman Measures Up* (Charlottetown, Canada: Ragweed Press, 1986), p. 50.

friend or a soft playground for any exploring love."* The qualities
that she loves about her fat self include a lot of those we normally
associate with being a teddy bear. She loves those. But that's exactly
what the other fat dyke doesn't want to be for anyone: "And I am
not your blasted teddy bear."

What, exactly, is a teddy bear? In the first place, teddy bears are
always fat. You never see a thin one. Sometimes they have lost their
stuffing, but new they are round and squeezable, carpeted and soft.
Often they are as big as the baby, and thus give shelter, warm embracing protection. They stand guard over the one they sleep with, they
intimidate strangers with their ferocity, these bears, but they are
infinitely forgiving, enfolding, enclosing, a playground, a pillow, a
friend.

You can love a fat person because they are a teddy bear, or even
a daddy bear.

There's a pornographic story in the big boy magazine called
Bulk Male. The new masseur meets his nine o'clock appointment:

> What stood before me was one of the most gorgeous men I
> had ever seen. He was about 6 feet tall, must have weighed in
> at about 350 lbs., had brown hair and blue eyes, and a beard
> with a mustache. . . . I tried not to get carried away with the
> mounds of flesh I found myself suddenly groping and grab-
> bing. . . . I paid special attention to those large round buttocks
> that screamed out to be squeezed.[†]

* *Fat Girl,* no. 3 (1995), p. 41.
[†] Scott Abbott, "The Fat Farm," *Bulk Male* 5, no. 2 (1995), pp. 3–4.

Call this another teddy bear fantasy, like so many of the personal ads in these zines: A beefy butt seeks top, burly man, a huge hunk of man with furry tummy, seeks husky, hunky, heavy men:

> Hump, butch bottom, cab driver, 5'9", 200 lbs. . . . seeks beefier, chunkier, stockier, butcher, daddy, son, bear or cub to service.[*]
>
> I know you're out there. . . . Around 6', 300 lbs., round face, hairy body, large tits, fat fingers, large butt and calves.[†]

Selena has a girlfriend who is one of those people who loses weight without even trying to. But she doesn't feel as good in her body when she is less fat. She likes the fat and wants to keep it. "She's putting heavy cream on her cereal and going, 'I'm cold. . . .' " The fat is warmth, the fat is insulation, but it is also the oily, glistening, creamy embrace that feels like love. Feeling fat she feels good, her fat is her mother, her earth mother, goddess body that takes care of her, that makes her feel fine. She loves her mother fat who loves her. So she pours on the cream and eats fat.

Max sees herself as "short . . . white . . . nerdy, I guess," and she's right. She weighs between 200 and 300 pounds. She has glasses and wears a baseball cap turned around, big fat arms and narrow shoulders, a large cotton sleeveless undershirt over immense jockey shorts. Her body is a poem of bloated succulence. She confesses to being in love with plants:

[*] Ibid., p. 54.
[†] Ibid., p. 55.

She says into the recorder,

> I love plants. Here's my one big chance to talk about it. I love
> plants. . . . I love to take care of them, I love to communicate
> with them, I love to figure out what they need, and watch how
> what you do affects the way they grow, and feel them when
> they're happy and fix them when they're sad. It's just so great.
> I'm totally removed from society and it makes me so happy.
> When I'm depressed that's what keeps me alive. I have a suc-
> culent garden growing in my bedroom. I have more than fifty
> varieties of succulent plants.*

You can't help wondering if she dares to eat a peach, any plants.
She's got to, unless she's carnivorous in order to avoid being vege-
tarian. But this fat woman is mother to her own plants, the generosity of her fertile embrace is extended to this succulent world
without society, with whom she communes in secret ways about the
mysteries of their growth and happiness. If fat is fertility, she fertil-
izes fatly the plants she loves with her loving attention. She feeds
the succulents; and succulent, they feed her. They help her up
when she's depressed and make her happy, as a fat piece of chocolate would.

In the *Bulk Male* community of fat men, bears and the men
who love them, a central issue is the question of gainers and encouragers. It concerns those men whose sexual predilections are particularly focused on deliberately gaining weight or encouraging others

---

* *Fat Girl*, no. 1 (1994), p. 19

to do so. In the personal ads of these male magazines, the number of men encouragers who are seeking gainers, or vice versa, is surprising, even astonishing. There's even a 900 number you can call, the "Gainer Fantasy Line," for people who "want to meet others who want to get bigger or get you bigger."

Here's one of the want ads:

> Ever fantasize about being fattened to massive, waddling proportions or about becoming a fattening coach who balloons an eager trainee into a waddling ball of fat or being part of a couple into mutual fattening? Let's explore our fantasies over the phone.*

"Waddling" seems to be the crucial term here, the verbal equivalent of whatever it is that turns these guys on. They love the waddle, the side-to-side movement of fat bodies on short legs. Fat fantasies of waddling flesh feed the erotic imagination of these men, who love the swaying rhythm of fat, and the jiggle—the jerky, gently, lightly moving that makes fat flop and fly.

This want ad is in search of gainers or encouragers, or people who love both. Perhaps the erotic pleasure, the pleasure of feeding or being fed, has its origins in some infantile fantasy or early experience of being attracted to fat men. That was the hypothesis of one pseudonymous writer, Averill Dupois, who recounts the result of a survey he took at an annual gathering of gay gainers and encouragers, called EncourageCon '95, whose slogan is "A Pigout in

* _Bulk Male_ 5, no. 2 (1995), p. 52.

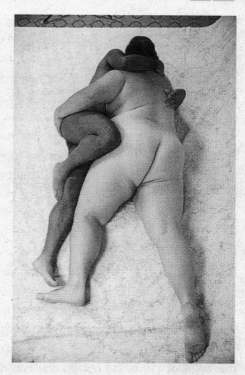

Fat love

Provincetown."* About a third of the men he interviewed had memories of positive attraction or intense identification with big-bellied men, "fat fathers or large-bellied uncles," or others who carried a significant amount of weight. One man told him of his "fascination" with the man's huge stomach and how he felt so protected "when he was held close to that big, round belly, and the

---

* *Big Ad*, no. 41 (August 1995), pp. 15–16.

pleasure he took in watching the man enjoy his food." Other com-
ments were "I worship bellies hanging out over the top of pants and
straining the shirt buttons on work uniforms such as those worn by
repair men." Another ad says, "Big belly, loves it and shows it whenever possible ISO other big-bellied guys to get together and pig out,
go to the beach and let everybody see how fat we are."*

I remember once sitting in a classroom in Paris listening to
Roland Barthes. He was a man of the most extraordinary taste, he
ate the most delicate food, and at that moment he was enormously
fat. I sat in front of the class and had a view of his enormous belly
pushing through the linen of his voluminous shirt. And I found
myself being affected and even aroused by a kind of aura or halo
that seemed to emerge from his paunch and suffuse it. I had never
had that experience before; it has happened since more than once.
But something like the mystic power of the belly is what you hear in
the want ads of these guys, in search of it. Belly worship is an old
story. It remains a very present one in the omnipresent figure of
Buddha, whose belly is the focus of the worshipers' gaze. There at
the navel of the globe resides the central point of energy from
which all his spiritual powers flow. The belly is itself a round mandala, a kind of prayer wheel, into whose entrancing convolutions
the celebrant dissolves.

Two thirds of the men interviewed at the EncourageCon '95
gathering had no particular memory of especially identifying with
or being attracted to fat men in their childhood. Maybe it's wrong to
suppose that what people remember and can recount about their

* Ibid., p. 16.

childhood has any more significance in their lives than what they may have experienced but repressed from memory. Rather than seeking psychological motives to explain encouragers and gainers, the love of fat bears, you could consider that it's an acquired taste. What sounds in our hemisphere like some kind of perversion might have a totally different meaning and value in another culture. Imagine that the following was an advertisement for sumo wrestlers, instead of a want ad in *Bulk Male*.

> Want to be bigger? To develop a gut, pecs, or ass to be envied? SO DO I! Let's work on increasing our bulk; if you're already there, how about giving out some pointers? Would you be interested in pigin' out and maybe working out? I'm forming a club for gainers and encouragers—supporting not only eating and other social events, but also body shaping (getting that fatter gut, pecs or ass), nutrition and other aspects of safe gaining. I'm 6', 240 lbs., 40″ waist, 50″ gut, br/gr, work in the computer industry and enjoy friends, fun, and fattening up.[*]

(I wish I knew exactly how he measures the difference between his waist and his gut.)

An American, David Benjamin, who writes about sumo wrestlers, takes it for granted that other Americans would find the big guts, fat asses, and thick thighs of these half-naked men to be repulsive. But he assures his reader that it's a taste he or she could learn to love.

[*] *Bulk Male* 5, no. 2, p. 44.

> Why do people keep coming back to contemplate those flanks
> of blubber—staring, judging? Well, because it's there. Fat is
> sumo's two-headed nickel, its flaw and its draw.... As you
> learn to live with it, you come oddly to appreciate it, but only
> with a conscious effort.°

Benjamin doesn't think that foreigners, particularly Americans,
could ever get to love this blubber, although you could oddly appreciate it. For Benjamin, that's as far as a white American could go in
developing a taste for what he takes for granted is disgusting. At the
same time, he thinks that a lot of the repulsion in America, the
fierce refusal even to look, is "secretly homophobic." His own story
takes him from ill-disguised disgust toward sumo fat, at the beginning of his book, to something like erotic love of it.

It's not the fat but the presence of so much undraped male flesh
that a lot of macho Americans, for example, don't want to let themselves look at. But even a tolerant American could never find these
bodies sexually desirable, and aesthetically beautiful the way, appar-
ently, a lot of Japanese women (no doubt some men) openly and
confidently do. Benjamin acknowledges that there is a Japanese aesthetic at work that is radically different from our own, one we can
oddly appreciate but never fully love.

> This is Japan, he writes, where the fat and the sylph-like, the
> whale and the butterfly, Audrey Hepburn and Meat Loaf,

° David Benjamin, *The Joy of Sumo: A Fan's Notes* (Rutland, Vt.: Charles E. Tut-
tle Co., 1991), p. 20.

share the same aesthetic universe and coexist in perfect harmony. The Japanese see little dissonance in aesthetic paradox, which is why a sumo wrestler usually marries a woman no larger than his right thigh.[*]

At the same time, Benjamin has been honest enough to explore the reactions of women who laugh when he speaks of the "unsightly fat" on sumo wrestlers. He adds, "In the sumo's nudity, women perceive softness, smoothness, sensuality, a huge, hairless, silky, breathing form upon which one can creep and climb, explore, taste and smell and probe and play out a whole anthology of larger-than-life sexual imaginings"[†] The desire to touch the blubbery flesh of these men, to fondle and press this fat, leads to pleasure, Benjamin recalls, like one Melville knew, and summons, homoerotically, in *Moby-Dick*, when the sailors are squeezing the precious oil out of great pieces of sperm whale blubber piled up on deck:

> Squeeze! squeeze! squeeze! all the morning long; I squeezed that sperm till I myself almost melted into it; I squeezed that sperm till a strange sort of insanity came over me; and I found myself unwittingly squeezing my co-laborers' hands in it, mistaking their hands for the gentle globules. Such an abounding, affectionate, friendly, loving feeling did this avocation beget; that at last I was continually squeezing their hands, and looking up into their eyes sentimentally; as much

[*] Ibid., p. 21.
[†] Ibid., p. 272.

to say,—Oh! my dear fellow beings, why should we longer cherish any social acerbities, or know the slightest ill-humor or envy! Come; let us squeeze hands all around; nay, let us all squeeze ourselves into each other; let us squeeze ourselves universally into the very milk and sperm of human kindness. Would that I could keep squeezing sperm for ever!°

Sumos are great whales whose fat one wants to squeeze. Benjamin, suffering from his own American fat phobia, speaks of sumo wrestlers as having "the endearing grace that fat men exude when they conquer the absurdity of their shape" (Benjamin, p. 199). Benjamin notes what is rarely observed: "we respond with incongruous esteem to those fat men whose suavity transcends their obesity."

Conquering and transcending obesity, some fatties achieve "suavity." *Suave* in Latin means "sweet; in English it's often a little too smooth and sweet. When fat gets suave, it accompanies a graceful gentleness of manner, a pleasing urbanity, beneath which the ridiculousness of fat vanishes. A suave sumo commands our fascinated look by his confidence in the pleasure he knows his fat procures for a dazzled audience of fans.

It's true that some fat people don't make us laugh. There is something charismatic about them that surrounds them with an aura not only of imposing gravity but irresistible charm. The charm of those fat people, the sweetness that lies beneath the flesh or in their abundance of flesh has moved us all. There's something

---

° Herman Melville, *Moby-Dick* (London: Penguin, 1986), p. 527; quoted in Benjamin, p. 273.

endearing in them, for all their impressive size, like the chubby thighs and chunky cheeks of our president.

Nobody laughed at Orson Welles or Louis XIV, Kate Smith or Bessie Smith. Pavarotti is taken very seriously, no less is Helmut Kohl. Jessye Norman or Julia Child, for all their wit, have a certain gravitas. When Elizabeth Taylor was fat she looked like Divine, but Divine, like Elizabeth or Roseanne, has a fat presence that doesn't quit.

I sat down with some people I know, a guy who is a gay fashion designer and a woman who is a size eighteen, BAT (big and tall) well-to-do, well dressed. Together we looked at some of the pictures of fat women in *Women En Large:*° What turned everybody off the most was the cellulite on the legs of some of the women—vast wattled thighs, bumpy with pods of fat cells beneath the skin. Instantly, they recoiled at the image of so much unstretched, uneven flesh. If the flesh is fat but firm, the effect can be different. No woman needs to be told what a horror cellulite can be. Seen on these immensely fat women it provokes the most violent reactions of distaste or uneasy, hysterical laughter. Why does mottled skin on thighs, the hills and valleys of cellulite, make it hard to look at these women, kill any erotic thought or defuse any feelings of pleasure at the spectacle?

But then you pick up an issue of *Plumpers and Big Women.* There are a lot of polemics in this magazine about who qualifies to be fat, who can be included within the "identity" which is being presented here for those who love it. I thought maybe plumpers

---

° *Women En Large: Images of Fat Nudes* (San Francisco: Books in Focus, 1994).

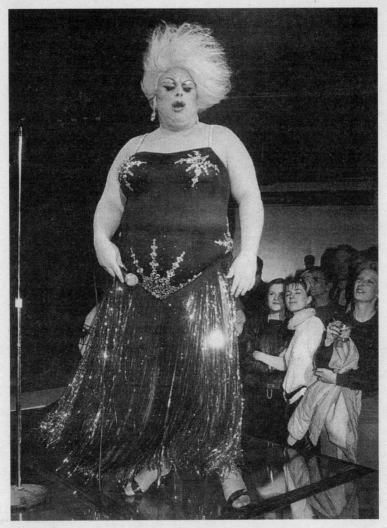

Divine

were the really, really big women, above, say, 225, where the super fat may begin. I called the editorial office, I explained my interest, and they told me they made no distinction between a plumper and a big woman. Plumpers sounds like Pampers, which is a kind of diaper. The words *plump* and *pamper* make you think those words might have some onomatopoeic origin, as if at the origins of language the sounded *mp* was fat. Consider primped and pumped, and frump, hump, and bump.

But then you look, say, at Teighlor—one of the real stars of the fat porn business at this moment. At 5'6" and 512 pounds, she

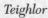

Teighlor

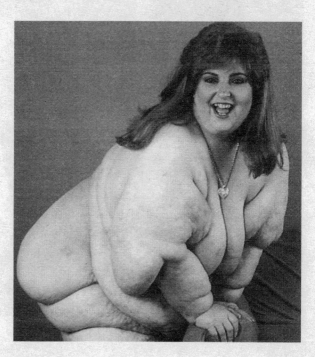

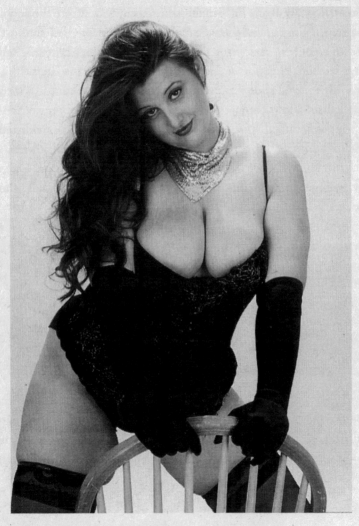

Woman in black

greatly outweighs her colleagues and competitors in commanding the passionate attention of her many admirers. At 512 she's way down from her max, which was 719 pounds. In her "early life," she was a model for Sears and weighed 103. "Then somewhere in there I started putting on weight." The readers of *Plumpers* think she is the queen of big women.

It is interesting to compare heterosexual *Plumpers* with *Fat Girl*. One dykes magazine is in color, the other in black-and-white; one is glossy, the other is air-brushed crass and in your face. One is pornographic, depicting available women (in Greek, *pornos* means harlot)—who sell their body or its image; the other is obscene, revealing things tabooed, visions of what ought not come to light. According to one historian, Veronique Nahoum, from the end of the Middle Ages until the nineteenth century people celebrated at essentially two kinds of parties. There were mostly rural festivals and popular feasts where people let themselves go, where they forgot their bodies, and partied hard. Then there were urban balls, upper-class receptions, where people were extremely conscious of how they looked, and their looks were shaped and colored and dressed to conform to a rigid ideal of beauty—oppressed by "the tyranny of a coded social image."[*] The women in *Plumpers* pose before the camera, they see themselves being seen, as if they were in front of a mirror. The pictures in *Fat Girl* don't appear for the most part to be posed, even if they were; they look as if these were women caught in the act of being fat, performing sex acts. The

---

[*] Veronique Nahoum, "La belle femme, ou le stade du miroir en histoire," *Communications* 31 (1979): 23.

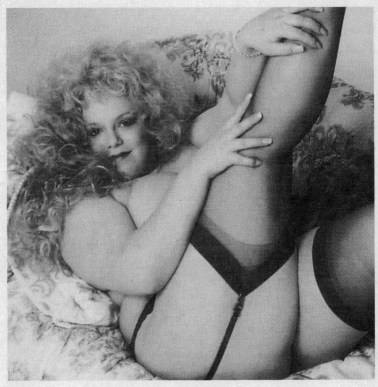

Gabrielle

women in *Plumpers* assume lascivious poses in front of the camera; they are being photographed not to record the mere fact of their size or the nature of their pleasure, but in order to excite the viewer. They are conscious of being very beautiful in the eyes of the camera, before the eyes of their admirers.

The women in *Plumpers* are the objects of a presumably heterosexual look, your average macho guy who happens to like his ladies big. The eyes scoping the fat dykes in *Fat Girl* have a totally different agenda for seeing. In the first case, the women are candy to the eye, conventionally posed in order effortlessly to be consumed by a viewer who already knows what he wants to see. With *Fat Girl,* you expect to be astounded. This zine represents a real breakthrough for fat. Even if it doesn't turn you on, it reveals the possibility of transvaluing the value of fat, of imagining new ways in which fat could once again become the focus of our erotic lives— the fleshy figure we most desire and find fabulous.

POLIT- ICAL FAT

Fat and politics is a subject that can be divided in two. On the one hand there is the question of the relation of obesity to particular economic or political circumstances. Germany after the war promoted fat and got fat. For a long time the Japanese, who for decades had little to eat, admired fat, and the erotic attention they devote to their sumos is an old and persistent tradition. There are those historians, like Hillel Schwartz, who go beyond the simple evidence that obesity is prized in periods following scarcity. They've argued in detail that the fattening of the population coincides with different stages in the development of capitalism. Fat in the population is a sort of sign, an index of the way capital is being formed.

On the other hand, you have the question of fat politicians, throughout history, rulers and presidents whose fat has served to

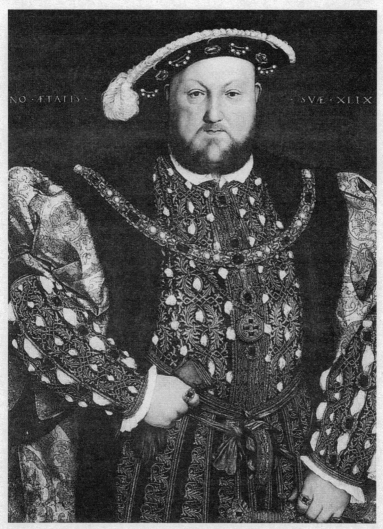

Henry VIII

impose themselves more forcefully on the world. Nero, Louis XIV, William Howard Taft, Churchill, Kohl, Clinton, on his good fat days (Newt Gingrich on his bad fat ones). These are big guys, bulk males, daddies of epic girth and political persuasion. They are men whose fat gives them presence and substance; lends to the aura of their personality the weight of importance, even a hint of intimidation.

It was reported last April that Clinton had put on a lot of weight, more than sixteen pounds since the previous years. Despite the best efforts of his wife, Hillary. She is very well known for the discipline she exercises over her own palate, and she views with alarm, which is both political and personal, the excess to which her husband is prone. He has at times enormous cravings, and pictures in the press of Clinton's fat or his eating create the impression of someone out of control. For Hillary Clinton, as for most of us, eating is a moral issue. A president, she fears, who can't command his own fat can't command.

There's a scene in *Primary Colors* where the first-lady character, who is keyed to Hillary Clinton, is in charge of snacks at the governor's mansion:

> "No more doughnuts," she said, carrying a bowl of bleached white popcorn over to the counter. "This is now the official snack food of the campaign. Henry, you eat this stuff—you lose weight. It has negative calories."[*]

Referring to the president, the First Lady in the novel adds, "He'll go for anything, if you provide it in sufficient quantity."

[*] Anonymous, *Primary Colors* (New York: Random House, 1996), p. 199.

It was reported that one evening Clinton and Kohl finished off, by themselves, an entire dessert cart at a fashionable Washington restaurant. It is probably true that in some future administration the real secret life of Clinton will be revealed. We will learn what the press probably knows but doesn't advertise. Its silence represents a form of respect for the taboo against showing or being seen eating in public. It's like the way the press handled Kennedy's affairs. Today they wouldn't hesitate to reveal sexual peccadilloes, but how many people know that when Hillary is away the amount of pizza delivered to the White House increases by 18 percent? Who do you think is eating those extra pies? Why don't we ever see Bill on TV gulping down hamburgers, as he has been known to do, devouring them in great number at campaign stops in roadside diners? The press feels authorized to reveal every personal secret of a politician, but it would be overstepping some boundary of what was acceptable to show the president making a pig of himself.

The president's weight gain in 1994 came at the end of a year that was stressful not only politically. It was recorded a year after his wife, the First Lady, had summarily fired the white house chef, Chambertin, and banished his sauces, the whole repertory of his classic French cuisine. In his place she installed a whole other sort of cook, a little-known chef from a well-known health spa in West Virginia. Whereas before the prez was served his chicken demideuil drenched in truffled cream sauce, now he got his fish simply grilled and accompanied with greens. The result of this new discipline exercised over his eating was that he gained a significant amount of weight. According to the necessity we have already many times observed: putting strict restrictions on your diet will ultimately result in your gaining more weight.

But the larger question is the role of fat in the political fortunes of President Clinton. While one can appreciate Hillary's concern for her husband's health and fortune, in these fat-phobic times we can't help wondering if she hasn't missed the point. Hillary Clinton encouraged her husband to get fat by discouraging him from eating what he loved. But getting fatter, he has also become more successful, more impressive, more of a leader. Journalists have suggested that Clinton's eating is a response to stress, which seems plausible. In the days following the Republican legislative triumph, he ate for consolation. And how he can eat! In a cookbook of the president's favorite recipes, written by his former statehouse chef (if that's what they call the cook in Arkansas), Clinton is particularly fond of beef chunks marinated in bottled Italian salad dressing and a frozen dessert made with Jell-O, whipped cream, and 7-Up. Pizza, hamburgers, and fried chicken are what gets him through some nights. And fritters. "Danny, where are those fritters?" asks the soon-to-be-president in *Primary Colors:*

> "Here, Governor," Danny offered them up front. "You know you're getting too fat to be a corpse."
>   "Fatten me up for the kill," [the governor] said. "Least I won't die hungry."*

We've already seen how powerfully food affects moods and compensates, often too well, for shifts in the body's chemistry. Fat food, junk food lift those endorphins and boost production of serotonin, and it makes even presidents, especially this one, feel good.

* Ibid., pp. 158–59.

You could consider the junk that Clinton consumed to be a form of self-medication, a kind of food therapy he practices to help him through difficult times. It's probably an old story with Clinton, the device and defense of a fatherless kid, who early on used food to reinforce his upbeat, optimistic personality when it was battered by loss and betrayal. Fat food makes Bill feel fine, puts the red in his cheeks, and fuels the enormous energy he draws upon to pursue his political ambitions.

There is some indication that putting on weight is the way Clinton fortifies his sense of solidity, virility, importance, and power. That seems certainly to have been the case with our fattest president, William Howard Taft. His biographer Judith Icke Anderson reports, for example, that after he was defeated for president by Professor Wilson of Princeton, President Taft became a professor at Yale. Within eight months of assuming his chair in New Haven, Taft went from 350 pounds, what he weighed at the end of his presidency, to 270. Relieved of the burdens of office, he relieved himself of eighty pounds and fired his valet, since now he could dress himself and tie his own shoelaces.* When Taft arrived at Yale, special accommodations were required. The distinguished chair he occupied had to be enlarged to oblige the swollen proportions of his presidential behind. When he was offered the Kent Chair of Constitutional Law, he replied that "it would not be adequate, but that perhaps a 'sofa of law' would do."† Special robes had to be sewn, since none of the standard sizes sufficed to drape his massive frame.

---

* Judith Icke Anderson, *William Howard Taft: An Intimate History* (New York: W. W. Norton, 1981), p. 256.

† Ibid., p. 256.

But eight months later, he had lost most of it, more quickly and more successfully than ever before in his life. Much of the weight he lost he had put on after he entered the White House and began eating "as never before," says Anderson. She gives us an example of one of Taft's "little" meals, as reported by a housekeeper. The meal included "lobster stew, salmon cutlets with peas, roast tenderloin with vegetable salad, roast turkey with potato salad, cold tongue and ham, frozen pudding [just like Clinton], cake, fruit and coffee."[*]

Taft's wife, Nellie, just like Hillary Clinton, assumed the duty of managing his diet in the White House. Her failure was a further source of political and personal anxiety. Her hectoring goaded Taft into escaping as often as he could from Washington and his "persecutors." He would summon his private train and escape to the countryside, far from public view, where he could eat to his heart's content. The train groaned beneath the burden of the presidential avoirdupois and the vast provisions, mounds of delicacies he had brought aboard.

One of the consequences of his fat was his tendency to fall asleep, particularly after meals, during meetings convened to do the most important business of government. The president frequently dozed over affairs of state. His wife called him "Sleeping Beauty." He replied to her, imperturbably, "Now, Nellie, you know it is just my way." He may have been right. There is some reason to think that successful presidents are those who sleep the most during their administrations. The "wisdom" of Ronald Reagan, for example, may have lain in his frequent dozing. Disinclined by his

[*] Ibid., p. 29.

slim genes to be fat, he nevertheless ate very well (no plain broiled fish at his table), drank wine, and slept through some of his most important briefings. Much of what a president is forced to hear is the noise of clashing self-interests. Maybe those who succeed are those who nod off, catching only fragments of what their chattering advisers say, half-sleeping, daydreaming their way toward some vision of the possible, unconsciously calculating the odds of achieving some defining political aim. If the most successful presidents were the ones who fell asleep the most over business, Jimmy Carter, I'll bet, was an insomniac.

> [President Taft's] face was wreathed in smiles, newsmen noticed, when on his first Thanksgiving Day in office he received a giant turkey from Rhode Island poultry men, a fifty-pound mincemeat pie from New York bankers, and a twenty-six-pound possum from Georgia, reputed to be the largest ever shot in the state. Guests present at the feast recounted that Taft sat back after his prodigious meal, smiled broadly, and said, "Thank goodness, I've had a dinner at which I haven't been compelled to make speeches. I've enjoyed food—real food—and I haven't had to work for it. [Anderson, pp. 125–26]

I'll bet that President Clinton understands what President Taft meant by real food. It's what he goes for when the going gets tough. It is food in such abundance, and of such richness, that it consoles the abysmal burdens of office, where the president never gets a free lunch, where everything he receives is paid for by the constant drain on his resources. Real food gives him unbounded, generous love, love that doesn't stop, doesn't ask for anything in return, a gift that keeps on giving and persists on the lips and the hips.

You may have seen the picture of Senator Dole lying out in the Florida sun wearing only a T-shirt and a bathing suit. He looked pretty good for a man of his age, pretty thin and trim for seventy-seven. If President Clinton were lying in the sun, there would be a lot more flesh to observe. Since he's younger and he runs, he must be in a lot better shape than Dole; Clinton must actually be harder, tougher, even if he has a lot of fleshy fat. Coming to the end of this book, six months before the presidential elections, I'd like to make a prediction. I predict, for all the reasons we have tried to suggest, that fat will be making a comeback, and if that's true, it should follow from that, as a general rule, in elections all over the world, as we approach the millennium, that the fattest man or woman will most always win. You mark my words; and if I'm right, will you EAT

FAT?

POST-SCRIPT

With the sort of irony that reinforces my belief in the unconscious, as I was writing this book, I was confronted in my personal life with a drama surrounding fat, which contradicts my book's conclusions. My mother had become so fat that it pressed on her lungs while she slept. In certain positions, her breathing, during sleep, was so inhibited that she entered apnea—the state of being breathless. At that moment the body, alarmed, caused her to wake briefly, until she shifted herself into a position that allowed her to sleep again, only to be awakened a little later. The effect of this breathless sleep is that she was tired all day long. Her fat was suffocating her. The more tired she became, the less able she was to find the energy to exercise her will, let alone to exercise. She was otherwise basically healthy and alert for a woman of her age, but her fat was weighing her down to the point of provoking immobility. At this moment in her life, according to her doctors, fat was her greatest enemy.

How could I tell my Mother, EAT

FAT? That's the last thing she needed. It felt as if, in her person, she had deconstructed my whole argument in this book. I had to admit that under these circumstances, the most responsible thing I could do as a son was to say to my mother, EAT

RICE. Our family considered sending her to Duke, where they have the famous rice diet weight-loss center. For, despite all her efforts, despite all the constant encouragement she received, the scoldings that rained down on her head, despite the diets and the doctors, the pills and the pep talks, despite her worsening apnea, she couldn't stop eating fat.

My mother believed, or so it seemed to me, in a magic bullet. She was persuaded that a pill or a procedure must exist, or would shortly, to relieve her of her fat. That's rather like an alcoholic who believes that at any moment he'll stop drinking. From constant dieting, my mother had gotten to the point where she was suffocating in fat. She had lost control of what was left of her control over eating. Now, when she needed to stop, she didn't seem to be able, not by herself. Unlike other kinds of addiction, eating is a habit one cannot renounce. Alcoholics can stop drinking; foodaholics can't swear off food, for very long. Every day, with every mouthful, the question of eating or not eating gets decided in favor of the former.

When fat becomes medically dangerous, and weight loss becomes a matter of life and death, eating rice is the equivalent of going on the wagon. It is not even strictly a diet. The word *diet* comes from the Greek *dieta*, which at its root probably comes from the word *zoein*, to live—a way of life. Eating only rice is the emblem of eating reduced to its minimal necessary condition, more like fasting—no way to live at all. If ghosts eat, they eat rice. Sometimes, in order to live, it may be necessary to eat like you're already dead. There are times when it seems like the only thing that protects you against death is dying.

But then I told my mother about Dr. Levitsky.

David Levitsky, Ph.D., is a professor of nutrition and psychology at Cornell, and one of the leading researchers on obesity in America. He is the author of a well-known study, whose conclusions dispute those of Dr. Manson. In *Malnutrition and Behavior: New Perspectives,** he demonstrated that increased mortality among non-smokers who were immoderately thin—their rate of early death—was equivalent to that associated with the very fat. According to Dr. Levitsky, it's entirely possible to be too thin. His own position toward fat is admirably tolerant, even while he is impressed by its role in increased heart disease, diabetes, and cancer.

In a recent editorial in the *Ithaca Journal*[†] he points out that the scientific literature "clearly has shown" that although some fat people may eat larger meals, they eat fewer meals. Their average calorie intake therefore is not necessarily different from that of thinner people. They may not move around as much, but because of their size the fat expend no less total energy than the thin. Furthermore, he cites evidence that

1. While certain kinds of pathologies—hypertension, hyperlipidemia, and diabetes—occur more frequently in groups of large people, most large people do not suffer from

* David Levitsky, Ph.D., *Malnutrition and Behavior: New Perspectives* (Ithaca, N.Y.: Cornell University Press, 1979).

[†] *Ithaca Journal,* October 17, 1995.

these pathologies and are as healthy as their thinner counterparts.

2. Fat people can "substantially reduce their risk [from these pathologies] by losing as little as 10 percent of their weight as a result of moderate changes in diet and exercise."

So I said to my mom, You got to exercise and change your diet. Otherwise you won't be able to breathe. Losing 10 percent of her fat sounded do-able. She did it. She started to exercise, four or five times a week at the Heart Center, and with her friends at the pool. She changed her diet. Started eating fruit. She lost 19 pounds, 10 percent of her weight. She suddenly had energy, she was sleeping through the night. She could move, she could walk, even hurry again. A new woman. She's still fat, but it's not morbid. She still looks beautiful, and now she looks healthy. She's happy. It's a blessing we owe to Dr. Levitsky.

FAT FAT FAT
FAT EAT FAT EAT
FAT FAT FAT FAT FAT
EAT FAT EAT FAT EAT
FAT FAT FAT FAT
FAT FAT
FAT FAT FAT FAT FAT
EAT FAT EAT FAT EAT
FAT FAT FAT FAT FAT FAT
EAT FAT EAT FAT EAT FAT EAT
FAT FAT FAT FAT FAT FAT FAT FAT
EAT FAT EAT FAT EAT FAT EAT
FAT FAT FAT   FAT FAT FAT
FAT EAT FAT EAT FAT EAT FAT EAT FAT
EAT FAT EAT FAT EAT FAT EAT FAT EAT FAT
FAT FAT FAT FAT FAT FAT FAT FAT FAT FAT FAT FAT
FAT FAT FAT FAT FAT FAT FAT FAT FAT FAT FAT FAT
FAT EAT FAT EAT FAT EAT FAT EAT FAT EAT FAT EAT FAT
EAT FAT EAT FAT EAT FAT EAT FAT EAT FAT EAT FAT EAT
FAT EAT FAT EAT FAT EAT FAT EAT FAT EAT FAT EAT FAT
FAT FAT FAT FAT FAT FAT FAT FAT FAT FAT FAT FAT
FAT FAT FAT FAT FAT FAT FAT FAT FAT FAT FAT FAT
FAT EAT FAT EAT FAT EAT FAT EAT FAT EAT FAT
FAT FAT FAT FAT FAT   FAT FAT FAT FAT FAT
FAT FAT EAT FAT FAT   FAT FAT EAT FAT FAT
FAT FAT FAT FAT FAT   FAT FAT FAT FAT FAT
FAT FAT FAT FAT   FAT FAT FAT FAT
FAT EAT FAT EAT   EAT FAT EAT FAT
FAT FAT FAT FAT   FAT FAT FAT FAT
FAT EAT FAT   FAT EAT FAT
FAT FAT FAT   FAT FAT FAT
FAT EAT FAT   FAT EAT FAT
FAT FAT   FAT FAT